HEALTH CARE IN TRANSITION

CAREGIVING

PERSPECTIVES, EXPERIENCES AND CHALLENGES

HEALTH CARE IN TRANSITION

Additional books and e-books in this series can be found on Nova's website under the Series tab.

HEALTH CARE IN TRANSITION

CAREGIVING

PERSPECTIVES, EXPERIENCES AND CHALLENGES

STEFANO ELEUTERI
EDITOR

nova
Medicine & Health
New York

Library of Congress Cataloging-in-Publication Data

ISBN: 978-1-53616-889-1

Published by Nova Science Publishers, Inc. † New York

Contents

PREFACE

A caregiver (usually also known as informal caregiver) is an often unpaid and without formal training (in the related disease) member of a person's social network who helps them with activities of daily living. Caregiving is most commonly used to address impairments related to old age, disability, a disease, or a mental disorder.

Typical duties of a caregiver might include taking care of someone who has a chronic illness or disease; managing medications or talking to doctors and nurses on someone's behalf; helping to bathe or dress someone who is frail or disabled; or taking care of household chores, meals, or processes both formal and informal documentation related to health for someone who cannot do these things alone.

With an increasingly aging population in all developed societies, the role of caregiver has been increasingly recognized as an important one, both functionally and economically. Caregiving reflects various possible experience with potentially infinite perspectives. Many organizations which provide support for persons with disabilities have developed various forms of support for carers as well. However, different challenges for this category of people are still strong: it involves changes within the family system, and some caregivers may not possess the necessary resources to deal with caregiving demands. Many caregivers assume the caregiver role with little or no preparation and have to learn to deal with several aspects of care in a very short time. Literature shows that informal caregivers tend to experience more depressive symptoms and poorer physical health outcomes in comparison to non-caregivers. Moreover, informal caregivers have been repeatedly acknowledged as a model of chronic stress, due to the high level of daily stress that caregivers experience.

All of these changes may lead to a set of biopsychosocial disorders named as *burden*, that would result from the obligation to provide care, specifically within the context of a chronic or long-term disease. Caregiver burden has been conceptualized using a multidimensional perspective, in terms of physical, emotional, social and financial difficulties/problems experienced by the caregiver.

In this state of the art, this book aims to present some challenges caregivers may encounter during their role, suggesting also some possible perspectives useful for clinicians to address the different experiences of informal caregivers, also connected to the different pathologies the patients they care to suffer from and to the different relationships they have with them.

The first chapter of the book is devoted to the theme of burden and posttraumatic growth in adult caregivers of patients with cancer. Caring for someone with cancer can be a traumatic experience since the cancer diagnosis can lead to a significant amount of distress. Many studies have shown that caregivers of patients with cancer can experience higher levels of anxiety, depression and poor quality of life, and that these levels are equal or even greater than those found in patients. Nevertheless, more recently, studies have also shown that not only patients, but also their caregivers are able to experience positive changes in their lives as a result of this traumatic event. In this chapter, the authors aimed to characterize a sample of adult caregivers of patients with cancer by examining the associations between caregivers' sociodemographic (gender) and patients' clinical variables (length of patients' disease and treatment as well as the level of patients' dependency) and psychological variables (caregiving burden and posttraumatic growth), and the associations between burden and posttraumatic growth. Participants were 214 adult children caregivers of parents with cancer (74% women; Mean age = 33.12; SD = 9.15), and completed a Sociodemographic and Clinical Questionnaire, the Burden Assessment Scale, and the Posttraumatic Growth Inventory. Overall, disrupted activities were associated with a greater appreciation of life, guilt was associated with more changes in relating to others, and overall burden was associated with more changes in relating to others. Moreover, women caregivers who reported to provide care for less than 1 a year, whose parents' disease duration was less than 1 year, and those who perceived their parent as completely dependent on their caregiving experienced more burden but also more posttraumatic growth. These exploratory findings suggest that caregivers may experience burden when they care for a relative with cancer, but they are also able to experience growth, especially in the way they relate with others and appreciate life. Moreover, the results may help to identify caregivers who are greater risk for developing burden or may have more difficulties in experiencing growth and for this reason are likely to benefit more from psychosocial interventions.

In the second chapter, the authors reflect in an important topic concerning depression and its correlates in non-professional female caregivers of persons in a situation of dependency. It is known that care is a task assumed mostly by women. Given the great intensity and dedication the care situation demands, this group is especially vulnerable to the development of depression. This study aimed to analyze the sociodemographic characteristics of informal caregivers in Galicia with respect to the care situation and their clinical characteristics, discover the prevalence of Major Depressive Episodes (MDE) in this sector of the population, and examine the relationship between MDE and the sociodemographic characteristics of caregivers and care recipients, the care situation, and caregivers' clinical characteristics (burden, social support, and self-esteem). The final sample consisted of 448 informal caregivers in Galicia. The presence of MDE was evaluated using the Structured Clinical Interview for Axis I of the DSM-IV - Clinical Version (SCID-CV). 9.8% of participants met the criteria for currently experiencing an episode of major depression. No significant differences in depression prevalence were found in terms of age, marital status, social class, educational level, area of residence, employment, or household income. Caregivers who were burdened (adjusted OR = 3.87, 95% CI [1.62-9.25]), who had low levels of social support (adjusted OR = 2.94, 95% CI [1.45-5.98]), and who had low self-esteem (adjusted OR = 2.85, 95% CI [1.42-5.73]) were at an increased risk for depression.

In chapter three, the authors approach the theme around costs derived from caregiving. Being a non-professional caregiver is associated with negative consequences at different levels. Providing care has adverse effects on physical and mental health, resulting in considerable use of health services. However, caregivers also often suffer difficulties in achieving optimal performance in their paid and unpaid work. Despite these important repercussions, research on the costs related to the use of health services in this population is inconclusive. Similarly, there is hardly any data on the costs derived from impaired labor productivity as a result of health problems in caregivers. The objective of this study was to determine the most frequent health problems experiened by non-professional caregivers and to evaluate the use of health services and its predictors, direct medical costs, and indirect costs due to the loss of labor productivity. Trained psychologists collected information directly related to the study objectives from a random sample of 585 caregivers (86.8% women, mean age = 55.5 years) and administered the Trimbos/iMTA questionnaire for Costs associated with Psychiatric illness (TiC-P) to evaluate the use of medical resources and lost productivity at work. 70.6% of caregivers had used a health service in the previous three months. The services employed by the greatest proportion of caregivers were primary care physicians (59.1%), specialists (28.7%), allied health professionals (14.4%), and social workers (13.3%). The presence of chronic diseases or conditions (OR = 6.45) and symptoms of depression and anxiety (OR = 1.03) were significantly associated with an increase in the probability of using a health service. The average cost of medical services consumed, per caregiver, was €205.00 over the previous 3 months. Among caregivers with paid employment (n = 119), 16.8% were absent from work due to health problems for an average of 11.3 days in the previous month. Their reduced work efficiency resulted in a loss of 3.9 days of productivity in the previous month. This resulted in an average monthly cost of €66.47 for absences and €22.94 for reduced work efficiency per caregiver with paid employment.

The majority of caregivers used health services and a significant percentage of caregivers with paid employment saw their performance affected as a result of health problems. The costs of care, in terms of medical consumption and labor productivity, must be taken into account in health care policy planning.

Chapter four present a study carried out on educational courses for caregivers of older patients with hip fracture. Family caregivers' mental health is an important predictor of care recipients' institutionalization and a risk factor for care-recipient mortality. Caregiver burden and its associated stress negatively affect caregivers' perceived general physical and mental health and have been negatively correlated with the functional status of older adults family members after discharge following hip fracture surgery. The rehabilitation process is highly dependent on the quality of care provided by the family caregiver. hip fracture is considered an acute event and often caregivers do not have enough time to develop the necessary skills and competencies to provide adequate care. The literature shows that interventions improving social support for family caregivers of older adults were found to effectively increase caregivers' confidence, coping ability and caregiver outcomes. The aim of this chapter is to discuss the importance of educational courses as support for family members of older adults who have suffered a hip fracture and present the results of a recent study we have carried out. The study was carried out on 398 caregivers of patients with hip fracture (mean age: 46.2, from 28 to 69 years). They were administered educational courses, consisting of 12 hours of frontal presentations and 30 hours of teledidactics. Each participant was given a socio-demographic questionnaire and, at the baseline and post-hoc, the Caregiver Burden Inventory (CBI) and a questionnaire to assess knowledge on hip fracture. A questionnaire was also administered to assess their satisfaction on the intervention. 52% of our sample was composed of family caregivers, 89% were females and 92% had Italian citizenship. The mean caregiving period was 28 months, the mean age of patients was 81.92 years (from 72 to 99), with 88.4% of the patients being females. At the baseline, the mean knowledge score was 12.3/21, while after the intervention 18.2/21. The mean CBI score was 28.85 at the baseline and 26.4 after the intervention.

95% of participants declared to have a high level of satisfaction regarding the course. These findings confirm the usefulness of caregiver educational courses in order to decrease caregiver burden and implement knowledge on hip fracture. Trainings and support group interventions are needed to better prepare family caregivers to make decisions, to feel confident to be part of the health care plan of their dependent relative, to know their rights and services provider should encourage the family carers to take care of their physical and psychological needs as well.

In chapter five, the author reflect upon the importance of touch and contact within caring. Since the '60s, several studies have been showing the importance of touch, especially within the caring relationship and healthcare settings. Touch is the sense of reciprocity. Moreover, the interest in formal or informal caregivers' well-being and psychosocial functioning has already highlighted the fragility of this caring position. Since Touching is unavoidable in Caring, formal and informal caregivers might benefit from an implemented awareness of the impact of their touch style and way of they intend physical contact. In addition, caregivers' education has a pivotal role in reducing their burn-out and compassion fatigue. Thus it can be hypothesized a model of intervention (on social scale or family-oriented) to support who care for others that are living in a situation of frailty (such as: older citizens, persons with disability, end of life care and/or children) and help them to build together a corporeal vocabulary where the word Caring gain its original meaning back.

Chapter six focuses on caregivers of haemodialysis patients. Family caregivers play an important role in the support of dialysis people since they have poor physical status and difficulty in looking after themselves. Caregivers accompany patients to renal unit, manage complications of dialysis treatment, prepare patients' diet and help them with home activities.

However, family carers usually have physical and psychological burden, while they are disappointed due to the problems derived from this therapy. They usually have increased levels of anxiety and depression due to their bad financial situation, the severity of patients' pain, the long duration of hemodialysis and the old patient's age.

Additionally, those who live with dialysis people have limitations in their personal and social activities, while they often face difficulties with their job in order to look after their loved persons. Moreover, many caregivers feel anxiety about home haemodialysis, since they have to learn about new technologies and management of safety issues.

Thus, renal professionals need to provide family caregivers with effecting information and psychological support in order to improve their psychological status and the quality of their life.

Finally, in the last chapters, the authors present psychological, relational and sexual impact of caregiving partners with autoimmune rheumatic diseases:

Autoimmune diseases form a range of disorders from organ-specific to systemic disorders with multi-organ involvement. Rheumatic diseases touch all aspects of life and this includes, of course, the partner, with an impact on the relationship, on sexuality and reproduction. The aim of this chapter is to analyze the implications of caregiving a partner with an autoimmune rheumatic disease. Diseases will be separately studied, and a final recommendation will be included. Many factors connected to rheumatic autoimmune diseases may cause these patients to become dependent on other people. Increased knowledge and awareness of rheumatologists, nurses, and care providers about physical, sexual, and psychological aspects of care plays an important role in improved management of these patients.

Most patients with sexual dysfunction rarely talked about sexual complaints with their rheumatologist. The sexual health of patients with rheumatic diseases is often neglected, with the possibility for both patients and medical doctors to find it difficult to discuss about sex, in part also because effective treatment options are not still available.

Sexuality is influenced by physical and psychological consequences of rheumatic diseases, like depression, anxiety, negative body image, reduced sexual drive, hormonal imbalance, pain, fatigue, stiffness, functional impairment and side effects from treatments.

The common problem is communication, so an open conversation including inquiry about sexuality in routine care is the first step to improve the situation. To allow the patients to present problems and concerns without embarrassment is also important. After an open discussion is achieved, the treatment will depend on the specific patient's symptoms. However, there are some general recommendations including: discussion of the problems with the partner, principally about the partner's fear in causing pain or distress during sexual intercourse; exploring different positions; using analgesic drugs, heat, and muscle relaxants before sexual activity in order to decrease pain; exploring alternative methods of sexual expression; and physiotherapy.

A multidisciplinary approach is therefore essential, in order to provide prevention and care for their sexual life, providing a better quality of life both for these patients and their partners.

Stefano Eleuteri, PhD
Department of Psychology,
Sapienza University of Rome, Rome, Italy

In: Caregiving
Editor: Stefano Eleuteri

ISBN: 978-1-53616-889-1

Chapter 1

BURDEN AND POSTTRAUMATIC GROWTH IN ADULT CAREGIVERS OF CANCER PATIENTS

Ricardo João Teixeira[1], PhD, Tânia Brandão[2], PhD and M. Graça Pereira[3], PhD

[1]Department of Education and Psychology, University of Aveiro, Aveiro, Portugal;
Psychotherapy Department, Clínica da Ordem, Porto, Portugal;
IINFACTS Institute of Research and Advanced Training in Health Sciences and Technologies, Gandra, Portugal
[2]CIP – Department of Psychology, Autonomous University of Lisbon, Lisbon, Portugal; CPUP – Center for Psychology at University of Porto, Porto, Portugal
[3]School of Psychology, University of Minho, Braga, Portugal;
CIPsi – Psychology Research Center, University of Minho, Braga, Portugal

Abstract

Caring for someone with cancer can be a traumatic experience since the cancer diagnosis can lead to a significant amount of distress not only for the patients but also for their caregivers. Indeed, many studies have shown that caregivers of patients with cancer can experience higher levels of anxiety, depression and poor quality of life, and that these levels are equal or even greater than those found in patients. Nevertheless, more recently, studies have also shown that not only patients, but also their caregivers are able to experience positive changes in their lives as a result of this traumatic event. In this chapter, we aimed to characterize a sample of adult caregivers of patients with cancer by examining (1) the associations between caregivers' sociodemographic (gender) and patients' clinical variables (length of patients' disease and treatment as well as the level of patients' dependency) and psychological variables (caregiving burden and posttraumatic growth), and (2) the associations between burden and posttraumatic growth. Participants were 214 adult children caregivers of parents with cancer (74% women; Mean age = 33.12; SD = 9.15), and completed a Sociodemographic and Clinical Questionnaire, the Burden Assessment Scale, and the Posttraumatic Growth Inventory. Overall, disrupted activities were associated with a greater appreciation of life, guilt and burden were associated with more changes in relating to others. Moreover, women caregivers who reported to provide care for less than 1 a year, whose parents' disease duration was less than 1 year, and those who perceived their parent as completely dependent on their caregiving experienced more burden but also more posttraumatic growth. These exploratory findings suggest that caregivers may experience burden when they care for a relative with cancer, but they are also able to experience growth, especially in the way they relate with others and appreciate life. Moreover, the results may help to identify caregivers who are at greater risk for developing burden or may have more difficulties in experiencing growth and for this reason are likely to benefit more from psychosocial interventions.

Keywords: caregiving; cancer; posttraumatic growth

INTRODUCTION

Burden in Adult Children Caregivers in Oncology

In the last decades, the health care system of various countries has suffered a set of changes that contributed to add value to the informal caregivers as important resources for caring with patients with chronic diseases, especially patients with cancer (Ducharme et al., 2006). In fact, Stetz and Brown (2004) highlighted the important role of family members as a source of caregiving in the context of cancer, since improvements in medical treatments have contributed to higher cancer survival rates. For this reason, the family is confronted with a greater involvement in the care of their ill family member.

The informal caregiver is someone who provides unpaid and untrained care to someone close (often a family member) with a chronic illness or a debilitating disease (Kuster & Merkle, 2004). It is estimated that, in Europe, about 10% to 25% of the total population are informal caregivers (European Commission, 2018). Thus, nowadays, informal caregivers are considered an important element of the healthcare system worldwide, with both economic and social value. For instance, in terms of economic value, the value of the services provided by the informal caregivers was estimated at $470 billion in 2013 (The National Alliance for Caregiving and the Public Policy Institute, 2015). The Portuguese Association of Care (2016) estimated the value of the services provided by the informal caregivers at €4 billions per year.

The greater involvement of caregivers in patient's care contributed to an increase in caregiver's psychological distress given their lack of preparation, both instrumentally and emotionally. Indeed, caring for a family member can be particularly challenging, since it involves changes within the family system, and some caregivers may not possess the necessary resources to deal with caregiving demands. Many caregivers assume the caregiver role with little or no preparation and have to learn to deal with several aspects of care in a very short time (Eleuteri, Bellanti & Falaschi, 2016). The cancer diagnosis brings with it changes in the frequency and nature of the family's routines and rituals as well as in the roles, responsibilities and skills of family members (Crespo et al., 2013; Pereira & Lopes, 2002; Walczak, McDonald, Patterson, Dobinson, & Allison, 2018). Literature shows that informal caregivers tend to experience more depressive symptoms and poorer physical health outcomes in comparison to non-caregivers (Pinquart & Sörensen, 2003; Schulz & Sherwood, 2008; Vitaliano, Zhang, & Scanlon, 2003). Moreover, informal caregivers have been repeatedly acknowledged as a model of chronic stress, due to the high level of daily stress that caregivers experience (Eleuteri et al., 2018).

All ~~of~~ these changes may lead to a set of biopsychosocial disorders named ~~as~~ *burden*. The concept of burden in caregivers of patients with a mental illness was developed by Grad and Sainsbury in 1966 to describe all the negative consequences experienced by a family member of an ill patient. The burden would result from the obligation to provide care, specifically within the context of a chronic or long-term disease (Chou, 2000). Thus, family burden has been conceptualized, using a multidimensional perspective, in terms of physical, emotional, social and financial difficulties/problems experienced by the caregiver (Lidell, 2002; Yeh, Johnson, & Wang, 2002). Some authors, however, have proposed a dichotomized view of burden (Hoenig & Hamilton, 1966). In this sense, burden could be experienced in an objective or subjective way. According to Hoenig and Hamilton (1966), objective burden would be associated with the events or activities that contributed to the negative experience of caregiving, while subjective burden would be associated with the feelings resulting from the tasks as caregivers. Chou (2000) highlights a broader view of burden, stating that "it is a mediating force between the patient's impairment and the impact that caregiving has on the lives of the caregivers and their families" (p. 398). The assessment of burden in cancer caregivers is a high priority since it can affect the possibility to address patients' needs as well as the quality of the support provided and the relationship between patient and caregiver (Deeken et al., 2003).

The way caregivers deal with their role can be influenced by several factors. Yeh et al. (2002) emphasize two factors: (1) the prior relationship between the caregiver and the care recipient and (2) the characteristics of both parties. Deeken et al. (2003) emphasized the role of caregiver's personality, social support, family's functional status, and competing commitments as "filters" in the association between caregiving and burden, justifying the individual variability in the way caregivers experience or not burden.

When the caregivers are adult children, the difficulties faced by them may be even higher. They have to balance their responsibilities as spouses or parents and as employees, along with their responsibilities as caregivers. Studies have shown that, after parental cancer, these caregivers tend to feel more tired in their jobs, experiencing more concentration difficulties, more absenteeism, and more insecurity with regards to their professional future (Stetz, 2003). This overloading can contribute to impair their ability to provide an adequate support to their ill family member and can contribute to heighten the patient distress. Specifically, Deeken et al. (2003) stated that, when caregivers experience higher levels of burden, patients tend to experience unmet needs (Kristjanson & Ashcroft, 1994; Oberst, Thomas, Gass, & Ward, 1989).

Overall, women assume the main role as caregivers and are strongly involved in the informal support provided to the ill family member (Kim, Baker, Spillers, & Wellisch, 2006; Kim & Given, 2008). Actually, these women have been coined in the literature as the "sandwich generation" representing "adult children of the elderly who are sandwiched between their aging parents and their own maturing children (…) a segment of the population roughly between 45 and 65 years of age" (Miller, 1981, p. 419). Studies have shown that adult children caregivers of patients with cancer that have children (18-64 years) tend to experience higher levels of burden, in comparison to adult children caregivers of patients with cancer without children. Moreover, studies have shown that female employed women tend to balance their multiple responsibilities by giving up of their leisure time (Stephens, Townsend, Martire, & Druley, 2001) or by reducing their paid hours or even by leaving their jobs (Enright & Friss, 1987; Raveis et al., 1999) in order to maintain the time of care provided to their ill family member.

Posttraumatic Growth and Caregiving in Oncology

The experience of caregiving for a parent with cancer has been examined especially in terms of negative outcomes (e.g., anxiety, depression, distress, burden). More recently, however, there has been an increased interest on the positive outcomes. Joseph and Linley (2008) argued that posttraumatic stress and posttraumatic growth could be conceptualized using a single framework. According to Cordova (2008), the following cancer characteristics provide an opportunity for growth: the threat of death and the confrontation with mortality, the disruption of life because of cancer treatments, and the need for physical and emotional support. Cancer would be conceptualized as a "psychosocial transition" that shatters individuals' world basic assumptions and requires the development of new skills to deal with it (Janoff-Bulman, 2000 cited in Cordova, 2008). The term *posttraumatic growth* (PTG) was first proposed by Calhoun and Tedeschi (2004) to describe the positive and transformational psychological changes in individuals after struggling with a major life event. It would involve a "change in people that goes beyond an ability to resist and not be damaged by highly stressful circumstances; it involves a movement beyond pre-trauma levels of adaptation" (Tedeschi & Calhoun, 2004, p.4).

Studies have shown that both individuals and their family members are likely to experience PTG after cancer (e.g., Barakat, et al. 2005; Manne et al., 2004; Schulz & Mohamed 2004; Widows, 2005; Mosher & Danoff-Burg, 2006; Mystakidou et al., 2007). However, individual differences exist in the development of PTG. In a previous longitudinal study (Manne et al., 2004), the development of PTG in patients was associated with younger age, greater contemplating reasons for cancer and more emotional expression; partners' PTG was associated with younger age, more intrusive thoughts, and greater use of positive reappraisal and emotional processing. In a recent study with couples facing breast cancer, Ávila, Coimbra, Park, and Matos (2017) found that partners' attachment security was associated with PTG for both members of the couple highlighting the need of assessing the couple as the unit of analysis. In terms of parent-child relationship, one study found that about 93% of adult daughters reported at least one positive change in their lives after parental cancer (Leedham & Meyerowitz, 1999). In another study conducted with the daughters of breast cancer survivors, authors found ~~that~~ they reported higher PTG in comparison to women with healthy parents; and the factors associated with PTG among these women included: life satisfaction, social support, emotional processing strategies, and problem-focused coping strategies (Mosher & Danoff-Burg 2006). These results are in accordance with the model proposed by Calhoun and Tedeschi (2008): some individual factors (such as optimism and coping strategies) and some contextual factors (such as social support) facilitate the development of PTG. According to Mosher and Danoff-Burg (2006), having time to cognitively process the experience of cancer, especially in an emotionally supportive social context, would contribute to the development of PTG. In the same study, the authors also found that actively managing one's emotions and cancer-related stress was associated with the development of cancer, as predicted by Calhoun and Tedeschi's (1998) model. Thus, it seems that those women who tend to engage in more adaptive coping strategies (e.g., planning, active coping, seeking social support, and processing emotions) tend to report more PTG (Mosher & Danoff-Burg, 2006). It is important to note that in some studies with cancer patients, however, social support and optimism were not related to PTG (e.g., Cordova, 2008; Sears et al., 2003). The use of diverse resources to face the stressor (in this case, the cancer diagnosis) and the tendency to have an active role to deal with it seem to facilitate the development of PTG (Calhoun & Tedeschi, 1998; Mosher & Danoff-Burg, 2006).

More recently, using a sample of adult children caregivers facing parental cancer, Teixeira and Pereira (2014a) found that gender, education, disease duration, dependency, distress, and family flexibility predicted higher levels of PTG Psychological morbidity (namely, anxiety, depression, distress and PTSD) was positively correlated with PTG (Teixeira & Pereira, 2014b). In the same study, parental dependency was found to be an important variable since it was associated with higher levels of PTG.

In sum, there is evidence that PTG exists in the context of cancer, not only for patients but also for their caregivers. Also, there are some individual, event-related and contextual factors that contribute to hinder or facilitate the development of PTG within this context. The link between perceived burden and PTG, however, remains unexplored. The objective of the present study was study PTG by examining not only differences according to individual (gender) and event-related factors (length of disease, length of chemotherapy, and level of dependency) but also by exploring associations between PTG and burden.

Methods

Participants and Procedures

The sample consisted of 214 adult children of patients undergoing chemotherapy (all White). The sociodemographic and clinical data collected about parents was completed by their adult children. Of these, 74% were women, with a mean age of 33.1 years (SD = 9.1; range = 18–61 years); 47% had a partner; and 63% had less than a high school education. Concerning clinical information, 60% registered the disease duration of the parent as less than one year, 69% noted that the parent was on chemotherapy for less than one year, and only 39% provided care for more than one year. Only 21% of adult children perceived the parent in treatment as completely reliant on their caregiving. Of the parents, 57% were female, with an average age of 62.1 years (SD = 9.2; range = 42–85 years), and 78% were married. 60% of parents had cancer of the digestive system, 21% of the reproductive system, 7% in the respiratory system, and 12% in other areas.

This study is cross-sectional approved by the Ethics Committees of three general hospitals in the North of Portugal. Participants were adult children who, during the period of data collection, accompanied the parent diagnosed with cancer to chemotherapy. This study used a convenience sample with voluntary participation. Inclusion criteria were: age $\geq$ 18 years, having a parent (or both) in chemotherapy, accompany the parent to the hospital for treatment (minimum criterion for defining the adult children as "caregiver"), and not being diagnosed with an oncological, psychiatric, or neurological disease. All participants were invited to take part in the study, informed about its purpose, and were assured of anonymity and confidentiality.

Measures

Demographic and Clinical Questionnaire

This questionnaire recorded the demographic and clinical data related to adult children and their ill parent. Clinical data reflect actual information that adult children had access to. Concerning the assessment of parental dependency, two response possibilities were created ('relatively dependent' or 'dependent'), considering daily living activities. Therefore, when asked about parental dependency, adult children answers reflected their perception of caregiving's physical aspects.

Burden Assessment Scale (BAS; Reinhard, Gubman, Horwitz, & Minsky, 1994; Portuguese version by Cotrim, 2007)

This is a 19-item measure that evaluates burden in an objective way, that is, the amendment of caring for someone with limitations imposed on activities and resources of the caregiver. BAS uses a 4-point scale (1–4), with higher scores indicating greater levels of caregiving burden. The Cronbach's alphas for the subscales and total scale were as follows: a = 0.82 for limitation of activity, a = 0.64 for feelings of worry and guilt, a=0.71 for social burden, and a + 0.81 for the total scale.

Posttraumatic Growth Inventory (PTGI; Tedeschi & Calhoun, 1996; Portuguese version by Teixeira & Pereira, 2013)

Self-responses are organized on a 6-point scale (0–5), with higher values corresponding to greater PTG. Participants were asked to focus on the experience of caregiving for their parent with cancer. Pearson correlations between the subscales and the total score were high ($p < .001$), and Cronbach's alphas were .85, .84, .87, .69, and .62 for the new possibilities, personal strength, relating to others, spiritual growth, and appreciation of life subscales, respectively. Internal consistency of the global scale was .94.

Data Analysis

Descriptive statistics were obtained after ensuring that all variables followed a normal distribution. Group differences according to gender, length of disease, duration of chemotherapy and level of dependency on PTG and BAS dimensions were examined using multivariate analyses of variance (MANOVAs). In order to examine the differences on the global PTG and BAS analyses of variance (ANOVAs) were conducted. Pearson correlation was used to test the association between PTG and burden.

RESULTS

Descriptive Statistics

Descriptive statistics are presented in Table 1.

Table 1. Descriptive statistics for posttraumatic growth (PTG) and burden (BAS) subscales according to gender

	Men (n + 56)	Women (n + 158)	Total
	M (SD)	M (SD)	M (SD)
PTG (total score)	51.48 (19.85)	59.94 (22.26)	57.73 (21.93)
Relating to others	15.93 (7.06)	18.13 (7.10)	17.55 (7.14)
New possibilities	10.36 (5.67)	12.22 (6.36)	11.73 (6.23)
Spiritual growth	3.75 (2.77)	4.82 (3.33)	4.54 (3.22)
Appreciation of life	8.07 (2.83)	9.18 (3.35)	8.89 (3.25)
Personal strength	13.38 (5.94)	15.60 (5.72)	15.02 (5.85)
BAS (total score)	33.27 (7.18)	37.65 (8.51)	36.50 (8.39)
Limitation in activity	13.09 (4.13)	16.11 (5.37)	15.32 (5.23)
Feelings of worry and guilt	13.57 (3.42)	14.59 (3.63)	14.33 (3.59)
Social burden	6.61 (2.02)	6.94 (2.43)	6.86 (2.33)

Note. N = 214.

Group Differences

Gender

Significant gender differences were found for PTG (total score) (F (1) = 6.31, $p < .05$, $\eta^2 = .03$), PTG relating to others (F (1) = 3.97, $p < .05$, $\eta^2 = .02$), PTG spiritual growth (F (1) = 4.61, $p < .05$, $\eta^2 = .02$), PTG appreciation of life (F (1) = 4.93, $p < .05$, $\eta^2 = .02$), and PTG personal strength (F (1) = 6.13, $p < .05$, $\eta^2 = .03$). No differences were found for PTG new possibilities (F (1) = 3.73, *ns*). Significant gender differences were also found for BAS (total score) (F (1) = 11.83, $p < .01$, $\eta^2 = .05$) and BAS limitation in activity (F (1) = 14.63, $p < .001$, $\eta^2 = .07$). No differences were found for BAS feelings of worry and guilt (F (1) = 3.39, $p = .07$) and BAS social burden (F (1) = .86, $p = .36$). Means and standard deviations are presented in Table 1.

Disease Duration

Significant differences were found for PTG – appreciation of life (F (1) = 4.34, $p < .05$, $\eta^2 = .02$) and for BAS (total score) (F (1) = 10.04, $p < .01$, $\eta^2 = .05$) and BAS – limitation in activity (F (1) = 14.87, $p < .001$, $\eta^2 = .07$). No differences were found for the remaining dimensions: PTG (total score) (F (1) = 1.55, *ns*), PTG relating to others (F (1) = 1.82, *ns*), PTG new possibilities (F (1) = .131, *ns*), PTG spiritual growth (F (1) = .265, *ns*), PTG personal strength (F (1) = .136, *ns*), BAS feelings of worry and guilt (F (1) = .635, *ns*), and BAS social burden (F (1) = 2.43, *ns*). Means and standard deviations are presented in Table 2.

Chemotherapy Duration

Significant differences were found for PTG appreciation of life (F (1) = 6.32, $p < .05$, $\eta^2 = .03$) and for BAS limitation in activity (F (1) = 3.94, $p < .05$, $\eta^2 = .02$). No differences were found for the remaining dimensions: PTG total score (F (1) = 1.84, *ns*), PTG relating to others (F (1) = 1.01, *ns*), PTG new possibilities (F (1) = 2.38, *ns*), PTG spiritual growth (F (1) = .766, *ns*), PTG personal strength (F (1) = .112, *ns*), BAS total score (F (1) = 2.02, *ns*),

BAS feelings of worry and guilt (F (1) = .004, *ns*), and BAS social burden (F (1) = .307, *ns*). Means and standard deviations are presented in Table 2.

Table 2. Descriptive statistics for posttraumatic growth (PTG) and burden (BAS) subscales according to length of disease, length of care, length of chemotherapy, and level of dependency

	Disease < 1 year (n = 130)[a]	Disease > 1 year (n = 84)[a]	Chemo < 1 year (n = 120)[b]	Chemo > 1 year (n = 94)[b]	Low dependency (n = 169)[c]	High dependency (n = 45)[c]
	M (SD)	M (SD)	M (SD)	M (SD)	M (SD)	M (SD)
PTG (total score)	56.23 (21.96)	60.05 (21.81)	55.93 (21.70)	60.02 (22.12)	**55.09 (21.49)**	**67.62 (20.90)**
Relating to others	17.02 (7.39)	18.37 (6.70)	17.12 (7.28)	18.11 (6.95)	**16.65 (7.09)**	**20.96 (6.31)**
New possibilities	11.34 (6.10)	12.33 (6.41)	11.15 (6.04)	12.47 (6.41)	**11.07 (6.06)**	**14.20 (6.28)**
Spiritual growth	4.45 (3.26)	4.68 (3.17)	4.37 (3.27)	4.76 (3.16)	**4.14 (3.22)**	**6.02 (2.82)**
Appreciation of life	**8.52 (3.21)**	**9.46 (3.26)**	**8.40 (3.33)**	**9.52 (3.05)**	8.84 (3.17)	9.09 (3.56)
Personal strength	14.90 (6.19)	15.20 (5.31)	14.90 (6.08)	15.17 (5.57)	**14.40 (5.77)**	**17.36 (5.60)**
BAS (total score)	**37.93 (8.34)**	**34.29 (8.03)**	37.22 (8.54)	35.59 (8.14)	**35.27 (7.61)**	**41.13 (9.57)**
Limitation in activity	**16.39 (5.25)**	**13.65 (4.79)**	**15.94 (5.25)**	**14.52 (5.13)**	**14.66 (4.99)**	**17.80 (5.45)**
Feelings of worry and guilt	14.48 (3.49)	14.08 (3.76)	14.34 (3.43)	14.31 (3.81)	**14.02 (3.59)**	**15.49 (3.40)**
Social burden	7.05 (2.50)	6.55 (2.01)	6.93 (2.37)	6.76 (2.29)	**6.59 (1.98)**	**7.84 (3.16)**

Note. N = 214; [a]Disease duration, "0 = below one year" or "1 = above one year"; [b]Chemotherapy duration, "0 = below one year" or "1 = above one year"; [c]Level of parental dependency, "0 = relatively dependent" or "1 = dependent". Statistically significant differences are presented in bold.

Level of Dependency

Significant differences were found for PTG total score (F (1) = 12.21, $p < .01$, $\eta^2 = .05$), PTG relating to others (F (1) = 13.72, $p < .001$, $\eta^2 = .06$), PTG new possibilities (F (1) = 9.33, $p < .01$, $\eta^2 = .04$), PTG spiritual growth (F (1) = 12.77, $p < .001$, $\eta^2 = .06$), and PTG personal strength (F (1) = 9.46, $p < .05$, $\eta^2 = .04$). No differences were found for PTG appreciation of life (F (1) = .207, *ns*). Significant differences were also found for BAS total score (F (1) = 18.83, $p < .001$, $\eta^2 = .08$), BAS limitation in activity (F (1) = 13.57, $p < .001$, $\eta^2 = .06$), BAS feelings of worry and guilt (F (1) = 6.10, $p < .05$, $\eta^2 = .03$), and BAS social burden (F (1) = 10-74, $p < .01$, $\eta^2 = .05$). Means and standard deviations are presented in Table 2.

Correlations

Correlations among study variables are presented in Table 3. As expected, all the dimensions of the PTG were positively ~~significantly~~ associated with each other. The same happened with the dimensions of the BAS. PTG relating to others was positively associated with the BAS (total score) and with the BAS – feelings of worry and guilt. PTG appreciation of life was positively associated with the BAS – limitation in activity.

Table 3. Correlations among study variables

	1	2	3	4	5	6	7	8	9
1. PTG (total score)	-								
2. Relating to others	.918**	-							
3. New possibilities	.910**	.806**	-						
4. Spiritual growth	.722**	.598**	.593**	-					
5. Appreciation of life	.731**	.572**	.621**	.491**	-				
6. Personal strength	.855**	.716**	.692**	.520**	.554**	-			
7. BAS (total score)	.128	.149*	.115	.098	.110	.062	-		
8. Limitation in activity	.124	.092	.112	.083	.165*	.098	.831**	-	
9. Feelings of worry and guilt	.113	.169*	.091	.112	.081	.015	.721**	.297**	-
10. Social burden	.008	.071	.024	-.005	-.101	-.022	.622**	.287**	.386**

Note. N = 214; *p<.05; **p <.01.

Discussion

Studies have shown that a cancer diagnosis may have negative implications not only for the patients but also for their caregivers. More recently, however, studies have also examined the positive outcomes of cancer diagnosis among both patients and caregivers. The present study aimed to examine differences in terms of burden and PTG according to individual (gender) and event-related factors (length of disease, length of chemotherapy and level of dependency) and to explore the association between burden and PTG among caregivers of patients with cancer.

The results showed differences in terms of gender. Women tended to report more PTG but also more burden than men. These results are consistent with other studies in the context of cancer (e.g., Zwahlen, Hagenbuch, Carley, Jenewein, & Buchi, 2010) and with studies from the larger field of trauma and psychology (e.g., Chappell, Dujela, & Smit, 2015; Tedeschi & Calhoun, 1996). In terms of burden levels, this may happen because women usually spent more time on caregiving (European Commission, 2018). Possible explanations for this are linked to the societal and cultural demands for women to adopt the role of caregiver (Sharma, Chakrabarti, & Grover, 2016) and to the differences in terms of their labor market participation (European Commission, 2018). Other studies suggest that gender differences in terms of coping resources could help to explain gender differences in burden levels. Indeed, women are more likely to use emotion-focused or ineffective coping strategies, in comparison to men that tend to use more problem-focused or other effective coping strategies (Sharma et al., 2016). The use of more emotion-focused coping strategies, however, can contribute to their higher levels of PTG, as cognitive and emotional processes are essential to develop PTG after a seismic event (e.g., Lindstrom, Cann, Calhoun, & Tedeschi, 2013).

Differences according to event-related characteristics were found in terms of disease length, length of chemotherapy and level of dependency. Findings suggest that caregiving burden is higher in the initial/acute phase of the disease. Indeed, the 'entrance' in this life-changing event may evoke a disruption in daily life, feelings of worry and unpreparedness, as well as the development of new roles (Pellegrino et al., 2010) that all together can contribute to the development of more burden. As expected, burden is high for those caring for patients with higher levels of dependency. Patient's impairment is usually associated with more physical and emotional demands for the caregivers (e.g., Cameron, Franche, Cheung, & Stewart, 2002; Nijboer, Triemstra, Tempelaar, Sanderman, & van den Bos, 1999). It usually leads to a greater disruption in the caregiver's life leading to more negative consequences associated with the caregiving task. For instance, a dependent relative requires more time of care which reduces the time available for other activities (Nijboer et al., 1999).

Regarding PTG, longer disease duration and longer treatments were both associated with more growth. Indeed, PTG is a process that do not result directly from the trauma but from the process and restructuration of the individual's schemata (Tedeschi & Calhoun, 2004). For this reason, it requires time to emerge. The development of PTG could also be related to the process of adaptation to their role and to the disease itself (Cormio et al., 2014) after the initial demands of the disease. The perception of parents' dependency in the context of the cancer could be a strong stressor that could promote more PTG (Calhoun & Tedeschi, 2008).

Finally, in terms of correlations, some dimensions of burden were associated with some dimensions of PTG. PTG – relating to others was positively associated with the BAS (total score) and with the BAS – feelings of worry and guilt. Although no causal relationship can be drawn, this result seems to suggest that burden or distress may be needed for the development of PTG. Especially, in the context of cancer caregiving, burden or distress seem to contribute to changes in the experience of relationship with others. Indeed, cancer places a threat to the relationship with a significant person (the parents). The confront with the potential loss of the significant parental relationship could contribute to higher levels of burden and distress (especially at the initial phase of the disease) but also for the strengthening of a more positive and closer relationships with the parents (Taku et al., 2008; Tedeschi & Calhoun, 1996).

Also, BAS – limitations in activity was positively associated with more PTG – appreciation of life. This result seems to suggest that while caregivers experience limitations in personal actions and activities as a result of their role, it also contributes to change their general philosophy of life and basic life assumptions (Taku et al., 2008; Tedeschi & Calhoun, 1996). These associations between burden measures and PTG is not a surprise since

Calhoun and Tedeschi (2006) have highlighted the fact that a stressful situation may produce PTG, and also ~~to~~ produce significant distress. In fact, previous studies have shown that measures of distress and PTG coexist (e.g., Morris, Shakespeare-Finch, Rieck, & Newbery, 2005).

Limitations and Directions for Future Research

Results should be interpreted with caution given its limitations. First, the cross-sectional nature of this study does not allow to determine causality between burden and PTG. Future longitudinal studies should be conducted. Second, these results rely on self-report questionnaires. Future studies should include other type of informants (e.g., the patients) and other type of data collection (e.g., diaries). Third, given the voluntary participation of the sample, it is possible that those caregivers who accepted to participate are those who better adapted to their role of caregiver or to the disease. Finally, potential mechanisms linking burden and PTG were not explored; further studies are needed to better understand the process of PTG development.

References

Ávila, M., Coimbra, J. L., Park, C. L., & Matos, P. M. (2017). Attachment and posttraumatic growth after breast cancer: A dyadic approach. *Psycho-Oncology, 26*(11), 1929-1935. doi: 10.1002/pon.4409.

Barakat, L. P., Alderfer, M. A., & Kazak, A. E. (2005). Posttraumatic growth in adolescent survivors of cancer and their mothers and fathers. *Journal of Pediatric Psychology, 31*(4), 413-419. doi: 10.1093/jpepsy/jsj058.

Calhoun, L. G., & Tedeschi, R. G. (1998). Beyond recovery from trauma: Implications for clinical practice and research. *Journal of Social Issues, 54*(2), 357-371. doi: 10.1111/0022-4537.701998070.

Calhoun, L. G., & Tedeschi, R. G. (2004). Authors' response: "The Foundations of Posttraumatic Growth: New Considerations".

Psychological Inquiry, 15(1), 93-102. doi: 10.1207/s15327965pli1501_03.

Calhoun, L. G., & Tedeschi, R. G. (2008). The paradox of struggling with trauma: Guidelines for practice and directions for research. In A. P. Linley & S. Joseph (Eds), *Trauma, recovery, and growth: Positive psychological perspectives on posttraumatic stress* (pp. 325-337). Hoboken, NJ: John Wiley & Sons.

Cameron, J. I., Franche, R. L., Cheung, A. M., & Stewart, D. E. (2002). Lifestyle interference and emotional distress in family caregivers of advanced cancer patients. *Cancer, 94*(2), 521-527. doi: 10.1002/cncr.10212.

Chappell, N. L., Dujela, C., & Smith, A. (2015). Caregiver well-being: Intersections of relationship and gender. *Research on Aging, 37*(6), 623-645. doi: 10.1177/0164027514549258.

Chou, K. R. (2000). Caregiver burden: A concept analysis. *Journal of Pediatric Nursing, 15*(6), 398-407. doi: 10.1053/jpdn.2000.16709.

Cordova, M. J. (2008). Facilitating posttraumatic growth following cancer. In A. P. Linley & S. Joseph (Eds), *Trauma, recovery, and growth: Positive psychological perspectives on posttraumatic stress* (pp. 185-206). Hoboken, NJ: John Wiley & Sons.

Cormio, C., Romito, F., Viscanti, G., Turaccio, M., Lorusso, V., & Mattioli, V. (2014). Psychological well-being and posttraumatic growth in caregivers of cancer patients. *Frontiers in Psychology, 5*, 1342. doi: 10.3389/fpsyg.2014.01342.

Cotrim, H. M. (2007). *Impacto do Cancro Colorectal no Doente e Cuidadores/Família: Implicações para o Cuidar [Impact of Colorectal Cancer on the Patient and Caregivers/Family: Implications for Caring].* PhD Dissertation. Porto, Portugal: Instituto de Ciências Biomédicas Abel Salazar.

Crespo, C., Santos, S., Canavarro, M. C., Kielpikowski, M., Pryor, J., & Féres-Carneiro, T. (2013). Family routines and rituals in the context of chronic conditions: A review. *International Journal of Psychology, 48*(5), 729-746. doi: 10.1080/00207594.2013.806811.

Deeken, J. F., Taylor, K. L., Mangan, P., Yabroff, K. R., & Ingham, J. M. (2003). Care for the caregivers: A review of self-report instruments developed to measure the burden, needs, and quality of life of informal caregivers. *Journal of Pain and Symptom Management, 26*(4), 922-953. doi: 10.1016/S0885-3924(03)00327-0.

Ducharme, F., Lévesque, L., Lachance, L., Zarit, S., Vézina, J., Gangbè, M., & Caron, C. D. (2006). Older husbands as caregivers of their wives: A descriptive study of the context and relational aspects of care. *International Journal of Nursing Studies, 43*(5), 567-579. doi: 10.1016/j.ijnurstu.2005.07.007.

Eleuteri, S., Bellanti, G., Falaschi, P. (2016). Hip fracture: preliminary results supporting significant correlations between the psychological wellbeing of patients and their relative caregivers. *Journal of Gerontology & Geriatrics, 64*, 104-111.

Eleuteri, S., Norton, M.C., Livi, F., Grano, C., Lucidi, F., Violani, C., ... Lombardo, C. (2018) Sleep quality as predictor of BMI in non-depressed caregivers of people with dementia, *Eating and Weight Disorders*, 23(5), 553-560. doi: 10.1007/s40519-018-0560-8.

Enright, R. B., & Friss, L. (1987). *Employed caregivers of brain-impaired adults: An assessment of the dual role.* Family Survival Project.

European Commission (2018). *Informal care in Europe: Exploring Formalisation, Availability and Quality*. LSE Consulting.

Grad, J., & Sainsbury, P. (1966). Problems of caring for the mentally ill at home. *Proceedings of the Royal Society of Medicine, 59*, 20-23.

Hoenig, J., & Hamilton, M. W. (1966). The schizophrenic patient in the community and his effect on the household. *International Journal of Social Psychiatry, 12*(3), 165-176. doi: 10.1177/002076406601200301.

Joseph, S., & Linley, P. A. (Eds.). (2008). *Trauma, recovery, and growth: Positive psychological perspectives on posttraumatic stress.* John Wiley & Sons.

Kim, Y., & Given, B. A. (2008). Quality of life of family caregivers of cancer survivors: Across the trajectory of the illness. *Cancer, 112*(S11), 2556-2568. doi: 10.1002/cncr.23449.

Kim, Y., Baker, F., Spillers, R. L., & Wellisch, D. K. (2006). Psychological adjustment of cancer caregivers with multiple roles. *Psycho-Oncology, 15*(9), 795-804.

Kristjanson, L. J., & Ashcroft, T. (1994). The family's cancer journey: A literature review. *Cancer Nursing, 17*(1), 1-17.

Kuster, P. A., & Merkle, C. J. (2004). Caregiving stress, immune function, and health: Implications for research with parents of medically fragile children. *Issues in Comprehensive Pediatric Nursing, 27*(4), 257-276. doi: 10.1080/01460860490884165.

Leedham, B., & Meyerowitz, B. E. (1999). Responses to parental cancer: A clinical perspective. *Journal of Clinical Psychology in Medical Settings, 6*(4), 441-461. doi: 10.1023/A:1026228000254.

Lidell, E. (2002). Family support—a burden to patient and caregiver. *European Journal of Cardiovascular Nursing, 1*(2), 149-152.

Lindstrom, C. M., Cann, A., Calhoun, L. G., & Tedeschi, R. G. (2013). The relationship of core belief challenge, rumination, disclosure, and sociocultural elements to posttraumatic growth. *Psychological Trauma: Theory, Research, Practice, and Policy, 5*(1), 50-55. doi: 10.1037/a0022030.

Manne, S., Ostroff, J., Winkel, G., Goldstein, L., Fox, K., & Grana, G. (2004). Posttraumatic growth after breast cancer: Patient, partner, and couple perspectives. *Psychosomatic medicine, 66*(3), 442-454.

Miller, D. A. (1981). The 'sandwich' generation: Adult children of the aging. *Social Work, 26*(5), 419-423.

Morris, B. A., Shakespeare-Finch, J., Rieck, M., & Newbery, J. (2005). Multidimensional nature of posttraumatic growth in an Australian population. *Journal of Traumatic Stress, 18*(5), 575-585. doi: 10.1002/jts.2006.

Mosher, C. E., & Danoff-Burg, S. (2006). A review of age differences in psychological adjustment to breast cancer. *Journal of Psychosocial Oncology, 23*(2-3), 101-114. doi: 10.1300/J077v23n02_07.

Mystakidou, K., Parpa, E., Tsilika, E., Pathiaki, M., Gennatas, K., Smyrniotis, V., & Vassiliou, I. (2007). The relationship of subjective sleep quality, pain, and quality of life in advanced cancer patients. *Sleep, 30*(6), 737-742. doi: 10.1093/sleep/30.6.737.

Nijboer, C., Triemstra, M., Tempelaar, R., Sanderman, R., & van den Bos, G. A. (1999). Determinants of caregiving experiences and mental health of partners of cancer patients. *Cancer, 86*(4), 577-588.

Oberst, M. T., Thomas, S. E., Gass, K. A., & Ward, S. E. (1989). Caregiving demands and appraisal of stress among family caregivers. *Cancer nursing, 12*(4), 209-215.

Pellegrino, R., Formica, V., Portarena, I., Mariotti, S., Grenga, I., Del Monte, G., & Roselli, M. (2010). Caregiver distress in the early phases of cancer. *Anticancer Research, 30*(11), 4657-4663.

Pereira, M. G., & Lopes, C. (2002). *O doente oncológico e a sua família* [*The cancer patient and his family*]. Lisboa: Climepsi Editores.

Pinquart, M., & Sörensen, S. (2003). Differences between caregivers and noncaregivers in psychological health and physical health: A meta-analysis. *Psychology and Aging, 18*(2), 250. doi: 10.1037/0882-7974.18.2.250.

Raveis, V. H., Siegel, K., & Karus, D. (1999). Children's psychological distress following the death of a parent. *Journal of Youth and Adolescence, 28*(2), 165-180. doi: 10.1023/A:1021697230387.

Reinhard, S. C., Gubman, G. D., Horwitz, A. V., & Minsky, S. (1994). Burden assessment scale for families of the seriously mentally ill. *Evaluation and Program Planning, 17*(3), 261-269. doi: 10.1016/0149-7189(94)90004-3.

Schulz, R., & Sherwood, P. R. (2008). Physical and mental health effects of family caregiving. *Journal of Social Work Education, 44*(S3), 105-113. doi: 10.1097/01.NAJ.0000336406.45248.4c.

Schulz, U., & Mohamed, N. E. (2004). Turning the tide: Benefit finding after cancer surgery. *Social Science & Medicine, 59*(3), 653-662. doi: 10.1016/j.socscimed.2003.11.019.

Sears, S. R., Stanton, A. L., & Danoff-Burg, S. (2003). The yellow brick road and the emerald city: benefit finding, positive reappraisal coping and posttraumatic growth in women with early-stage breast cancer. *Health Psychology, 22*(5), 487. doi: 10.1037/0278-6133.22.5.487.

Sharma, N., Chakrabarti, S., & Grover, S. (2016). Gender differences in caregiving among family-caregivers of people with mental illnesses. *World Journal of Psychiatry, 6*(1), 7-17. doi: 10.5498/wjp.v6.i1.7.

Stephens, M. A. P., Townsend, A. L., Martire, L. M., & Druley, J. A. (2001). Balancing parent care with other roles: Interrole conflict of adult daughter caregivers. *The Journals of Gerontology Series B: Psychological Sciences and Social Sciences, 56*(1), 24-34. doi: 10.1093/geronb/56.1.P24.

Stetz, K. M., & Brown, M. A. (2004). Physical and psychosocial health in family caregiving: a comparison of AIDS and cancer caregivers. *Public Health Nursing, 21*(6), 533-540. doi: 10.1111/j.0737-1209.2004.21605.x.

Taku, K., Cann, A., Calhoun, L. G., & Tedeschi, R. G. (2008). The factor structure of the Posttraumatic Growth Inventory: A comparison of five models using confirmatory factor analysis. *Journal of Traumatic Stress, 21*(2), 158-164. doi: 10.1002/jts.20305.

Tedeschi, R. G., & Calhoun, L. G. (1996). The Posttraumatic Growth Inventory: Measuring the positive legacy of trauma. *Journal of Traumatic Stress, 9*(3), 455-471. doi: 10.1002/jts.2490090305.

Tedeschi, R. G., & Calhoun, L. G. (2004). Posttraumatic growth: Conceptual foundations and empirical evidence. *Psychological Inquiry, 15*(1), 1-18. doi: 10.1207/s15327965pli1501_01.

Teixeira, R. J., & Pereira, M. G. (2013). Factors contributing to posttraumatic growth and its buffering effect in adult children of cancer patients undergoing treatment. *Journal of Psychosocial Oncology, 31*(3), 235-265. doi: 10.1080/07347332.2013.778932.

Teixeira, R. J., & Pereira, M. G. (2014a). Family caregiver support to cancer patients: the relevance of adult children. In M. A. Paludi (Ed), *The Praeger Handbook on Women's Cancers: Personal and Psychosocial Insights: Personal and Psychosocial Insights* (pp. 305-334). California: ABC CLIO.

Teixeira, R. J., & Pereira, M. G. (2014b). Posttraumatic growth in adult children caregivers of cancer patients: contributing factors and processes. *Psycho-Oncology, 23* (S), 79-79. doi: 10.1080/07347332.2013.778932.

The National Alliance for Caregiving and the Public Policy Institute (2015). *Caregiving in the US – 2015 Report.* Retrieved from: https://www.aarp.org/content/dam/aarp/ppi/2015/caregiving-in-the-united-states-2015-report-revised.pdf.

The Portuguese Association of Care (2016). *Annual Report.* Retrieved from www.cuidadoresportugal.pt.

Vitaliano, P. P., Zhang, J., & Scanlan, J. M. (2003). Is caregiving hazardous to one's physical health? A meta-analysis. *Psychological Bulletin, 129*(6), 946-972. doi: 10.1037/0033-2909.129.6.94.

Walczak, A., McDonald, F., Patterson, P., Dobinson, K., & Allison, K. (2018). How does parental cancer affect adolescent and young adult offspring? A systematic review. *International Journal of Nursing Studies, 77*, 54-80. doi: 10.1016/j.ijnurstu.2017.08.017.

Widows, M. R., Jacobsen, P. B., Booth-Jones, M., & Fields, K. K. (2005). Predictors of posttraumatic growth following bone marrow transplantation for cancer. *Health Psychology, 24*(3), 266-273. doi: 10.1037/0278-6133.24.3.266.

Yeh, S. H., Johnson, M. A., & Wang, S. T. (2002). The changes in caregiver burden following nursing home placement. *International Journal of Nursing Studies, 39*(6), 59-600. doi: 10.1016/S0020-7489(01)00055-4.

Zwahlen, D., Hagenbuch, N., Carley, M. I., Jenewein, J., & Buchi, S. (2010). Posttraumatic growth in cancer patients and partners - effects of role, gender and the dyad on couples' posttraumatic growth experience. *Psycho-Oncology, 19*(1), 12-20. doi: 10.1002/pon.1486.

In: Caregiving
Editor: Stefano Eleuteri

ISBN: 978-1-53616-889-1

Chapter 2

DEPRESSION AND ITS CORRELATES IN NON-PROFESSIONAL FEMALE CAREGIVERS CARING FOR DEPENDENT PERSONS

Ángela Torres[1], PhD, Fernando Vázquez-Asper[1], Vanessa Blanco[2,*], PhD, Patricia Otero[3], PhD, Lara López[4], MD and Fernando L. Vázquez[4], PhD

[1]Department of Psychiatry, Radiology, Public Health, Nursing and Medicine, University of Santiago de Compostela, Santiago de Compostela, Spain

[2]Department of Evolutionary Psychology and Education, University of Santiago de Compostela, Santiago de Compostela, Spain

[3]Department of Psychology, University of A Coruña, A Coruña, Spain

[4]Department of Clinical Psychology and Psychobiology, University of Santiago de Compostela, Santiago de Compostela, Spain

* Corresponding Author's Email: vanessa.blanco@usc.es.

ABSTRACT

Informal care of dependents is a task assumed mostly by women. Given the great intensity and dedication the care situation demands, this group is especially vulnerable to the development of depression. However, few studies have used appropriate assessment instruments to determine the prevalence of depression in informal caregivers and its relationship with the sociodemographic characteristics of caregivers and care recipients, the specifics of the care situation, and the caregivers' clinical characteristics. This study aimed to: (a) analyze the sociodemographic characteristics of informal caregivers in Galicia (Spain) with respect to the care situation and their clinical characteristics, (b) discover the prevalence of Major Depressive Episodes (MDE) in this sector of the population, and (c) examine the relationship between MDE and the sociodemographic characteristics of caregivers and care recipients, the care situation, and caregivers' clinical characteristics (burden, social support, and self-esteem). The final sample consisted of 448 informal caregivers in Galicia. The presence of MDE was evaluated using the Structured Clinical Interview for Axis I of the DSM-IV - Clinical Version (SCID-CV). 9.8% of participants met the criteria for currently experiencing an episode of major depression. No significant differences in depression prevalence were found in terms of age, marital status, social class, educational level, area of residence, employment, or household income. Caregivers who were burdened (adjusted OR = 3.87, 95% CI [1.62-9.25]), who had low levels of social support (adjusted OR = 2.94, 95% CI [1.45-5.98]), and who had low self-esteem (adjusted OR = 2.85, 95% CI [1.42-5.73]) were at an increased risk for depression.

Keywords: informal caregiver, women, sociodemographic and care-related variables, burden, social support, self-esteem, depression, predictors

INTRODUCTION

Contextualizing the Phenomenon of Dependence

Advances in nutrition and medicine have led to a significant increase in life expectancy, which—added to the decline in birth rates—have led to an unprecedented global shift in demographics characterized by a rapidly aging population, especially in developed countries. According to United Nations [UN] projections (UN Department of Economic and Social Affairs, Population Division, 2017), between 2017 and 2050 the cohort of people over 60 will grow more than any other age group, more than doubling its current size by 2050 (see Figure 1). In absolute terms, this sector of the population will increase from 962 million to nearly 2.100 billion over the course of less than half a century. In parallel, we are witnessing a process of *aging of the aging*—that is, an increase in the population of very elderly persons (more than 80 years old). This figure will triple between 2017 and 2050, from 137 to 425 million people worldwide.

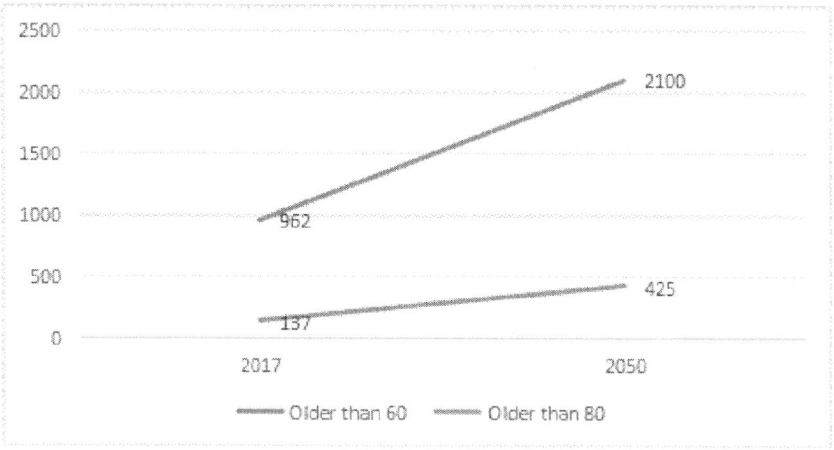

Figure 1. Increase in the worldwide population over 60 years old and over 80 years old between 2017 and 2050 (millions of people). Adapted from United Nations (UN) Department of Economic and Social Affairs, Population Division (2017).

At the same time, in the coming years, the number of people with disabilities or functional dependence will also follow an upward trend. Worldwide, the percentage of the lifespan lived with a disability increased from 21.1% in 1990 to 31.2% in 2013 (Vos et al., 2015), and it is estimated that by 2040 the number of dependent persons will increase by around 31% in developed countries. This increase will be as much as 60% in North America and Australia, and around 20% in Europe (Harwood, Sayer, & Hirschfeld, 2004).

Faced with such high numbers, social and health systems are insufficient to meet the daily needs of the dependent population. Thus, care for such persons must often be assumed by informal or non-professional caregivers, defined as people who provide help with personal care or activities of daily living to family members or friends with functional limitations (Colombo, Llena-Nozal, Mercier, & Tjadens, 2011; Feinberg & Pilisuk, 1999). Informal caregivers are part of the social network of persons with functional difficulties, so this type of care always involves a relationship of affection between the provider and the dependent person (García-Calvente, Mateo-Rodríguez, & Eguiguren, 2004; Jamieson, 1993) or at least a prior relationship with the other person. Caregivers may be relatives, friends, or neighbors, but most often a direct family member performs this role.

In OECD (Organization for Economic Cooperation and Development) countries, more than one out of every ten adults serve as a non-professional and unpaid caregiver (Colombo et al., 2011). Specifically, studies of caregivers in the United States point to figures of around 18 million people who assist older people with disabilities (Spillman, Wolff, Freedman, & Kasper, 2014), and 54.1 million persons providing care to persons over 18 years of age. This is equivalent to 24.1% of the adult population (National Alliance for Caregiving [NAC] and AARP Public Policy Institute [AARP], 2009). Various investigations at the international level find that the typical caregiver is female, middle-aged, married, without paid employment, the daughter or partner of the dependent person, taking care of another female over the age of 75 years, and providing between 1 and 8 hours of care daily (Colombo et al., 2011; National Alliance for Caregiving [NAC] and AARP Public Policy Institute [AARP] 2009; Pickard, 2011).

Studies in this field of research systematically confirm the existence of an overrepresentation of women in the role of informal caregiver (Colombo et al., 2011; Gallagher, Rose, Rivera, Lovett, & Thompson, 1989; NAC & AARP, 2009; Pickard, 2011), constituting about two-thirds of all such caregivers. Likewise, there are also differences by gender in the type of care tasks performed and in the intensity of the care provided. In general, women are responsible for care that requires greater daily dedication and a certain regularity in its provision (García-Calvente, Mateo-Rodríguez, & Maroto-Navarro, 2004;

Jenson & Jacobzone, 2000). Regarding the amount of time devoted to care tasks, female caretakers spend more hours per day providing care for the dependent person compared to male caregivers, and they do so for more years (García-Calvente, Del Río, & Marcos, 2011).

Table 1. Consequences of informal caregiving on caregivers' lives

Area		Repercussions
Social		Reduction of social interactions Abandonment of leisure activities Decreased time spent on self-care Social isolation
Family		Family conflicts for reasons related to care Less time spent with other family members (partner, children...)
Financial		Financial problems related to the expenses that care entails Conflicts over combining caregiving with work (need to reduce hours or even stop working) Decreased long-term job-related benefits
Health	Physical	Cardiovascular problems, immunological disorders, hormonal changes, infections, gastrointestinal disorders, bone and joint pain, excessive exhaustion and fatigue, sleep problems, sexual dysfunction, allergies, headaches...
	Mental	High levels of stress, feeling burdened, reduced measures of subjective well-being, reduced perceived self-efficacy, personal dissatisfaction... Mood disorders (anxiety and depression)

Similarly, there are gender differences in the negative impact on various areas of informal caregivers' lives as a result of their care duties, especially those who are primary caregivers (Del Pino, Frías, Palomino, & Martínez-Riera, 2012) (see Table 1). Given their greater involvement and time commitment, women experience a greater number of stressors related to care and suffer more negative effects than men (Pinquart & Sörensen, 2006). In the social and family realm, the problems caregivers experience most frequently include reduction of social interactions, deterioration in family relationships, abandonment of leisure activities, decrease in time for self-care, and lower self-esteem (García-Calvente, Mateo-Rodríguez, & Maroto-Navarro, 2004; Washington et al., 2015). Likewise, women are forced to give up paid employment outside home more often than men do, and they have more limitations in their opportunities to advance in their careers

(Colombo et al., 2011; Lee & Tang, 2015). Consequently, the negative financial impact of care is more pronounced for women: in the short term, they experience a greater decrease in income, while in the long term they have access to a smaller number of social benefits (e.g., job-based retirement plans [Austen & Ong, 2013; Lee & Tang, 2015; Muller & Volkov, 2009]).

In line with the above, several studies suggest that female caregivers experience almost twice as many health problems as men (Dentinger & Clarkberg, 2002; García-Calvente, Mateo-Rodríguez, & Maroto-Navarro, 2004; Morgan, Williams, Trussardi, & Gott, 2016; Yee & Schulz, 2000). At a physical level, women more frequently develop physical symptoms and diseases associated with caregiving (see Table 1) and report higher levels of fatigue (Mittelman, Roth, Clay, & Haley, 2007; Schulz & Sherwood, 2008). With regard to emotional health, the impact is even greater. According to the available evidence, caregivers are at risk for psychological deterioration starting at 25 hours of care a week (Masanet & La Parra, 2011). In general terms, informal caregivers experience high levels of stress and burden, and experience a decrease in subjective measures of well-being and perceived self-efficacy (Blanco et al., 2019; Crespo & López, 2007; Del Pino et al. 2012; Pinquart & Sörensen, 2003, 2007; Vázquez, Otero, Blanco, López, & Torres, 2018). All this leads to feelings of dissatisfaction with oneself and one's life and makes caregivers a population especially vulnerable to the development of mood disorders, especially depression (Dentinger & Clarkberg, 2002). International estimates suggest that the prevalence of depression in informal caregivers ranges from 14% to 55% (Cohen et al., 1990; Cuijpers, 2005; Gallagher et al., 1989; Grunfeld et al., 2004; Redinbaugh, MacCallum, & Kiecolt-Glasser, 1995; Schulz, O´Brien, Bookwala, & Fleissner, 1995). Some studies indicate that the risk of developing most mental disorders is generally higher in women than in men (Seedat et al., 2009; World Health Organization, 2004) and that approximately half of female caregivers experience depression, versus one-third of male caregivers (Gallagher et al., 1989; Livingston, Manela, & Katona, 1996).

However, despite the fact that women usually are involved in informal care, the phenomenology of depression in informal caregivers has not been sufficiently investigated. In addition, most studies available on the prevalence of depressive symptoms in this population have limitations.

A significant number of these studies focus on very specific samples, especially caregivers of people with dementia, Alzheimer Disease, or cognitive decline (e.g., Joling et al. 2010, 2012; Mahoney, Regan, Katona, & Livingston, 2005), and as a result, it is difficult to generalize based on them. Moreover, many studies determine the prevalence of depression using self-reported symptom scales (Mahoney et al., 2005; Kim, Shaffer, Carver, & Cannady, 2014) instead of using explicit diagnostic criteria. In this way, they do not provide sufficient information to make a clinically sensitive and specific diagnosis of depressive disorder using standardized diagnostic criteria such as those included in the Diagnostic and Statistical Manual of Mental Disorders of the American Psychiatric Association (DSM) or the International Classification of Diseases from the World Health Organization (ICD). As a consequence of all this, the prevalence of diagnosable depressive disorders among informal caregivers has not been definitively determined.

Likewise, we must add that evidence regarding the relationship between depression and sociodemographic variables, related to the care situation and the caregiver's clinical situation is scarce and contradictory. A caregiver variable that has been related to depression in this population is age, but here the research has obtained contradictory results, with some studies finding greater depressive symptomatology in older caregivers (Jácome, Figueiredo, Gabriel, Cruz, & Marques, 2014; Koyama et al., 2017), and other studies finding higher rates of depression in younger caregivers (Blanco, Rohde, Vázquez, & Torres, 2014; Covinsky et al., 2003). A relationship has also been found between depression and being single (Derajew, Tolessa, Fevissa, Addisu, & Soboka, 2017). Higher levels of depression have been found in caregivers from the upper social classes (Blanco et al., 2014). Findings on educational level are not conclusive either, with depression being linked to higher levels of education in some studies (Argyriou et al., 2011), while others find a higher risk of developing depression in caregivers with a lower level of education (Covinsky et al., 2003; Lee, Lin, Chien, & Fang, 2015; Lu et al., 2007). With regard to area of residence, numerous studies agree that the burden of care—with everything that this entails—is greater among caregivers in urban areas (Bigbee, Musil, & Kenski, 2011; Imaiso, Tsukasaki, & Okoshi, 2012; Lee, Yoo, & Jung, 2010). In terms of job situation, a higher prevalence of depression has been found among unemployed caregivers (Lee et al., 2015). A greater risk for the development of depression has been found in lower-income caregivers (Majerovitz, 2007; Wang et al., 2016; Williams, Forbes, Mitchell, Essar, & Corbett, 2003). Looking at variables related to the care situation, the following have been considered to be risk factors for the development of depression: caring for a dependent person who is male or who is younger, being female, being the daughter of the dependent person (Covinsky et al., 2003; Pinquart & Sörensen, 2011; Chappell, Dujela, & Smith, 2015), and longer duration of care (Baillie, Norbeck, & Barnes, 1988; Guerriere et al., 2016) for more hours per day (Derajew et al., 2017; Yoon, Kim, Jung, Kim, & Kim, 2014). Other studies, however, have found no relationship between the duration of care and the development of depressive symptoms (Capistrant, Berkman, & Glymour, 2014). Regarding the illness of the dependent person, some researchers found lower subjective well-being in people providing care for children with mental illness or multiple disabilities (Hammond, Weinberg, & Cummins, 2014), those caring for people with cancer, dementia (Kim & Schulz, 2008), or with lower functional status (Guerriere et al., 2016). Other studies have found no differences in caregivers' depressive symptoms as a function of the cause of the care recipient's dependence (Crespo, López, & Zarit, 2005).

Finally, a relationship has also been found between depression and certain clinical variables of caregivers, such as burden, level of social support, and self-esteem. With respect to burden, some studies have found a relationship between the caregiver's burden and an increase in the likelihood of their developing depressive symptoms or even a depressive disorder (Epstein-Lubow, Davis, Miller, & Tremont, 2008; Gallagher, Phillips, Oliver, & Carroll, 2008; Grunfeld et al. 2004; Li, 2005; O'Rourke & Tuokko, 2004; Perlick et al., 2016; Tsai & Pai, 2016). An investigation (Thompson, Bundek, & Sobolew-Shubin, 1990) found that the association between burden and depression could be explained by other variables, such as the patient's physical deterioration, the quality of family relationships, and the caregiver's subjective interpretations. Some studies, moreover, have found social support to be protective against depression for caregivers (Ali & Kausar, 2016; Brummett, Siegler, Williams, Hilliard, & Dilworth-Anderson, 2012; Majerovitz, 2007; Pagel & Becker, 1987), while another work has found this effect only for certain types of social support, such as family support (Kuscu et al., 2009). In addition, a previous study (Casale, Wild, Cluver, & Kuo, 2015) found that social support protected against depression specifically in the female caregiver population. Low self-esteem has been considered a predictor of depressive symptoms in different samples of caregivers, while high self-esteem has been found to reduce the risk of depression in this population (Chung, Bakas, Plue, & Williams, 2016; Land, Hudson, & Stiefel, 2003; Zunzunegui, LlácerCentro, & Béland, 2002).

To conclude, an important additional limitation is that existing studies have focused on caregivers of both sexes and have not specifically analyzed the correlates of depression in the population of female caregivers, which is a much larger group in terms of informal care compared to men.

Objectives of the Study

This study sought to analyze the sociodemographic profile of caregivers and their clinical situation, and to examine the prevalence of major depressive episodes according to Axis I diagnostic criteria from the DSM-IV-TR and the associated variables (sociodemographic, care situation, and clinical variables) in a representative random sample of informal caregivers.

METHODS

Participants

A cross-sectional study of informal caregivers was carried out in Galicia, an autonomous community located in northwestern Spain, with an area of 29,434 km^2 and a population of 2,699,299 inhabitants. Caregivers had to meet a series of requirements for inclusion in the study: (a) be female; (b) be the primary caregiver for a dependent family member; (c) the care recipient was classified as dependent by the official agency; (d) the caregiver had to live in the same house as the person she cared for; and (e) the dependent person should not have a terminal prognosis with a timeline of less than 6 months. Those caregivers who did not give their consent were excluded from the study.

The study sample was taken from the database of informal caregivers registered in the official registry prepared by the Dependency Technical Coordination Unit of the Ministry of Labor and Welfare of the Autonomous Community of Galicia. This registry was created on the basis of Law 39/2006 of December 14, on the Promotion of Personal Autonomy and Care for Dependent Persons[1], in order to regulate the basic conditions of equality and attention for dependent persons.

Specifically, 478 caregivers were randomly selected from the database (precision of ±2 and confidence interval of 95%). Out of this initial sample, 30 candidates did not meet the eligibility criteria, leaving a final sample of 448 participants with an average age of 54.2 years ($SD = 10.5$; see Figure 2).

Caregivers were contacted personally by mail and telephone and invited to participate in the study after being informed of its nature, objectives, risks, and benefits. All participants gave their informed consent. Participation was voluntary and free, without any financial or other incentives. The study was carried out in accordance with the latest version of the Helsinki Declaration and obtained the approval of the bioethics committee at the University of Santiago de Compostela (Spain).

---

[1] Ley 39/2006, de 14 de diciembre, de Promoción de la autonomía personal y atención a las personas en situación de dependencia [Law 39/2006 of December 14, on the Promotion of Personal Autonomy and Care for Dependent Persons]. BOE 299 del 15 de diciembre del 2006. Retrieved from: https://www.boe.es/boe/dias/2006/12/15/pdfs/A44142-44156.pdf.

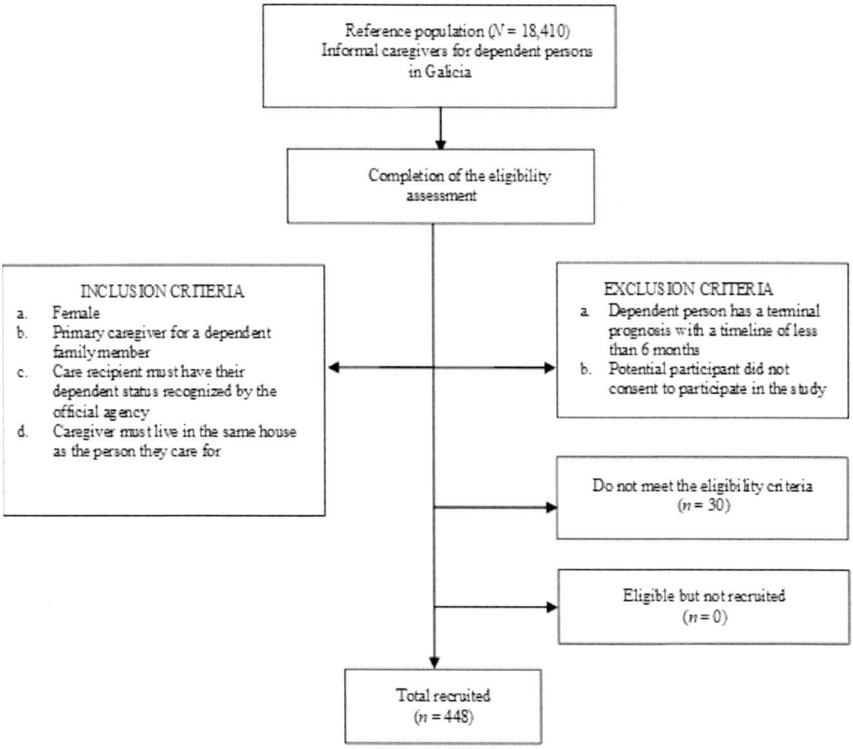

Figure 2. Flowchart of the study phases.

Instruments

Different instruments were used to gather information about the characteristics of the participants, the dependent person, the care situation, the presence of depression, levels of burden, perceived social support, and self-esteem.

An ad hoc questionnaire specifically developed for this study was used to collect sociodemographic data on the participant and the dependent person, as well as the characteristics of the care situation. This questionnaire included items about participants' age, marital status, social class, educational level, area of residence, employment status, and household monthly income. It also contained questions about the sex and age of the care recipient and about the illness that gave rise to their dependence. Regarding the care situation, information was gathered on the relationship between the caregiver and care recipient, duration (years of care), and intensity of care (daily hours). It should be noted that caregivers may provide informal help to one or more people; in such cases, the data collected refer to only one of them—specifically, to the one to whom the caregiver devoted the greatest amount of time or care because they are more dependent. The caregivers provided the information about the dependent persons they cared for.

The evaluators used the Spanish version of the Structured Clinical Interview for Axis I of the DSM-IV - Clinical Version (SCID-CV; First, Spitzer, Gibbon, & Williams, 1999) to determine the presence of a major depressive episode. The SCID-CV is a structured interview designed to provide information on the most common Axis I disorders in the DSM-IV, in a clinical setting. It consists of six modules, from A to F, which respectively address affective episodes, psychotic symptoms, psychotic disorders, mood disorders, substance-related disorders, anxiety disorders, and other disorders. Each item corresponds to a diagnostic criterion and has a classification of "+" or "–" depending on whether the diagnostic criterion is met; if it is doubtful, the category "?" should be indicated, and information should be collected to clarify whether this diagnostic criterion is met. SCID-CV scores are judgments about the diagnostic criteria and not necessarily the patient's answers to the questions. It is usually administered in a single session of 45 to 90 minutes. This diagnostic instrument is widely used and has been determined to be reliable, with Kappa values of .70 to 1.0 (First, Spitzer, Gibbon, & Williams, 2000).

The Caregiver Burden Interview (CBI; Zarit, Reever, & Bach-Peterson, 1980) was used to assess burden. The CBI consists of 22 items that evaluate the subjective burden associated with care, considering physical health and psychological well-being, economic situation, social relationships, and relationship with the care recipient, as well as one item on the global level of burden. Scores are given using a Likert scale of 0 (never) to 4 (almost always), with a total score that ranges from 0 to 88. There is a direct relationship between the score and the burden experienced by the caregiver.

Schreiner, Morimoto, Arai, and Zarit (2006) established a cutoff point of > 24, which correctly identified 72% of caregivers with probable depression. Several studies that have used this instrument report an internal consistency of between .79 and .92 (Neary, 1993). Specifically, this study used a translation into Spanish adapted to our environment and administered in accordance with Guillemin, Bombardier and Beaton's guidelines (1993), which included validation through back translation (Brislin, Lonner, & Thorndike, 1973); internal consistency was found to be satisfactory (Cronbach's $\alpha = .85$).

The Functional Social Support Questionnaire was used to evaluate social support (Duke UNC, Broadhead, Gehlbach, de Gruy, & Kaplan, 1988; Spanish version from Bellón, Delgado, Luna del Castillo, & Lardelli, 1996). This scale includes 11 items with a Likert scale response format ranging from 1 to 5. The total scale ranges from 11 to 55, and the higher the score the greater the social support perceived. Bellón et al. 1996 established a cutoff point that discriminated between low social support (<32) and normal social support (≥32). The internal consistency of the Spanish version of the scale was .90.

The Rosenberg Self-Esteem Scale (SES, Rosenberg, 1965; Spanish version from Fernández-Montalvo & Echeburúa, 1997) was used to evaluate self-esteem. This 10-item scale assesses self-esteem on a Likert scale that ranges from 1 (strongly agree) to 4 (strongly disagree). The total score ranges from 10 to 40. Higher scores correspond to higher self-esteem, with a cutoff point of 29 being established for the adult population (Ward, 1977). Its test-retest reliability is .85, and its internal consistency is .92.

Procedure

A research protocol was prepared detailing the objectives of the study, the design and the context, the participants (target population, accessible population, inclusion criteria, exclusion criteria, sampling, recruitment), measures (predictive and outcome variables), biases (non-response bias, recall bias, selection bias), data analysis strategy, quality control and data management, timeline, and ethical issues.

The evaluations were carried out by four psychologists with several years of experience (from 4 to 15 years) in the evaluation and diagnosis of mood disorders who had received specific training to evaluate the participants in this study. They received a full week of training before the study, including standard training components for the SCID-CV, the CBI, the Duke UNC and the SES, and they were supervised by two clinicians with an average of 20 years of experience in the evaluation and diagnosis of mental disorders, one of them affiliated with the Department of Clinical Psychology and Psychobiology at the University of Santiago de Compostela and the other with the Department of Psychiatry, Radiology, and Public Health of the same university.

After the research protocol was developed, a letter was sent to the informal caregivers inviting them to participate in the study, explaining what it consisted of, and indicating the date and place where they would be evaluated. Approximately two days before the scheduled date of the evaluation, they were contacted by telephone to remind them of the location, day, and time of the evaluation. Each participant was interviewed in person by the interviewers in a location near the address provided by the Dependency Unit of the Galicia Autonomous Government. The participants first answered questions about the sociodemographic characteristics of the caregivers, the care recipients, and the care situation, as described above. Then the evaluators identified the presence of depressive episodes using the SCID-CV. Finally, information on burden, social support, and self-esteem was collected through self-administered instruments. Each evaluation lasted approximately 60 minutes. One of the clinical experts supervised the interviewers weekly during the study. In addition, a random sample of 10% of the interviews was recorded and then analyzed by the other expert who supervised the training.

To minimize participant loss, some of the strategies recommended by Newman, Browner, Cummings and Hulley (2008) were followed, with special emphasis on treating study participants with kindness, friendliness, and respect, helping them to understand the research so that their participation in the study would be successful. Other strategies can be seen in Table 2.

Table 2. Strategies to reduce participant loss

A.	Schedule a systematic series of repeated contact attempts
B.	Reminders of the interview date
C.	Avoid invasive and annoying information-gathering procedures
D.	Present the study to participants in an attractive way

Data Analysis

All statistical analyses were performed using version 21.0 of the IBM SPSS Statistics statistical program. The following were considered when selecting the statistical tests: (a) the objective of the analysis, (b) the characteristics of the variables involved, (c) the specific conditions of each test, (d) the study design, and (e) the number of groups to be used.

First, different frequency analyses and descriptive statistics were performed to describe the characteristics of the caregivers, the care recipients, the care situation, and the clinical variables.

Bivariate logistic regression analyses were performed to examine the relationship between depression and each of the sociodemographic, care and clinical variables included in the study. Taking the statistical distribution as a reference (below or above the median). Some of these variables were first redefined into only two categories, being dichotomized as follows: participant age as ≤ 55 or > 55; care recipient age as ≤ 83 or > 83; and duration of care as ≤ 8 years or > 8 years. For statistical (given that people caring for their parents are the majority in this sample) and clinical reasons related to the findings of previous works that have found differences in terms of depression as a function of the relation to the person cared for (e.g., Covinsky et al., 2003), the kinship relationship was recoded as parent and other relationship. For statistical reasons (given that caregivers for persons with dementia are the majority in this sample) and clinical reasons related to the contradictory results in previous works that have assessed the consequences of caring for people with dementia versus other pathologies in terms of caregiver emotional state (e.g., Vázquez et al., 2018), the diagnosis of the care-recipient was recoded as dementia and not dementia. For clinical reasons, to distinguish care during daytime hours from care that exceeds those hours, daily hours of care were classified as $\leq$ 12 hours or > 12 hours per day. The clinical variables were dichotomized according to the cutoff point for the corresponding scale, yielding the following: burdened (CBI > 24) vs. not burdened (CBI $\leq$ 24); low social support (Duke UNC < 32) vs. normal social support (Duke UNC $\geq$ 32); and low self-esteem (SES $\leq$ 29) vs. high self-esteem (SES > 29).

Multivariate logistic regression analysis was then performed. Given the large sample size, a relaxed *p*-value criterion was used (as recommended by Sperandei [2014]), and all the variables with a $p \leq .30$ in the bivariate analyses were incorporated into the multivariate logistic regression analysis to determine the adjusted differences between the predictive variables and depression. The results were reported by providing adjusted odds ratios (OR) with 95% confidence intervals (CI). The sociodemographic variables for informal caregivers included in the analysis were age, marital status, social class, employment status, and cause of dependence. Finally, a relationship has also been found between depression and certain clinical variables in caregivers, such as feeling burdened, level of social support, and self-esteem.

Results

Characteristics of Informal Caregivers, Care Recipients, Care Situation, and Clinical Variables of Informal Caregivers

As shown in Table 3, 52.7% (n = 236) of the caregivers were under 55 years of age. The average age was 54.2 years (SD = 10.5), with a range of 21 to 84 years. Regarding caregivers, 76.6% (n = 343) were married or living as a couple, 50.9% (n = 228) belonged to the lower/lower-middle class,

Table 3. Characteristics of informal caregivers, care recipients, care situation, and clinical variables of informal caregivers

Variable	*n*	%
Age		
≤ 55 years	236	52.7
> 55 years	212	47.3
Marital status		
Single	105	23.4
Partnered	343	76.6
Social class		
Lower/Lower middle	228	50.9
Upper middle/Upper	220	49.1
Education level		
No schooling/primary school	378	84.4
Secondary education/university	70	15.6
Area of residence		
Rural	235	52.5
Urban	213	47.5
Employment situation		
Employed	72	16.1
Unemployed	376	83.9
Monthly household income		
< 1000 euros	111	24.8
≥ 1000 euros	337	75.2
Sex of the care recipient		
Male	122	27.2
Female	326	72.8
Age of the care recipient		
≤ 83	222	49.6
> 83	226	50.4
Relationship with the caregiver		
Caring for a parent	195	43.5
Caring for another person	253	56.5
Cause of dependence		
Dementia	182	40.6
Other diseases	266	59.4
Duration of care (years)		
≤ 8 years	222	49.6
> 8 years	226	50.4
Intensity of care (daily hours)		
≤ 12 hours	62	13.8
> 12 hours	386	86.2
Burden		
Burdened (CBI > 24)	231	51.6
Not burdened (CBI ≤ 24)	217	48.4
Social support		
Low social support (Duke UNC < 32)	121	27.0
Normal social support (Duke UNC ≥ 32)	327	73.0
Self-esteem		
Low self-esteem (SES ≤ 29)	137	30.6
High self-esteem (SES> 29)	311	69.4

84.4% (n = 378) had no education or had only completed primary school, and 52.5% (n = 235) lived in a rural environment. The majority (83.9%, n = 376) were unemployed, and the majority (75.2%, n = 337) stated they had a monthly household income of 1000 Euros or more.

Regarding the characteristics of care recipients, 72.8% (n = 326) were women; 50.4% (n = 226) were older than 83, with an average age of 74.2 (SD = 23.8) and a range of 2 to 104. With respect to the kinship relationship between the caregiver and the care recipient, the most frequent case was that the caregiver was caring for one of her parents (43.5%, n = 195); other caregivers (56.5%, n = 253) reported having another type of tie to the care recipient (caring for a partner/spouse, child, etc.). Regarding the cause of the care recipient's dependence, most caregivers indicated that their relative's dependence was due to dementia (40.6%, = 182). The remaining 59.4% (n = 266) indicated other diseases as the cause (e.g., cancer, musculoskeletal system diseases, or congenital diseases). In relation to the duration of care, 50.4% (n = 226) had provided care for their relative for more than 8 years; the average was 11.4 years (SD = 9.2), with a range of 1 to 47 years. Regards to the intensity of care, most caregivers provided more than 12 hours of care a day (86.2%, n = 386); the average was 16.6 hours devoted per day (SD = 3.5), ranging from 2 to 24 hours.

In relation to the clinical variables of caregivers, 51.6% (n = 231) were burdened, 73.0% (n = 327) had normal social support, and 69.4% (n = 311) had a high self-esteem.

Prevalence of Depression and Depressive Symptom Profile

According to the results of the SCID-CV, 9.8% (n = 44) of informal caregivers were experiencing a major depressive episode at the time of assessment.

It was found that the most frequent depressive symptoms in caregivers with depression were insomnia or hypersomnia and a decrease in the ability to think or concentrate (see Table 4). Both were experienced by 93.2% of caregivers with depression. To a lesser extent, although also at a high frequency, this group of caregivers reported depressed mood (84.1%), significant weight loss or gain (79.5%), psychomotor slowing or agitation (79.5%), recurrent thoughts of death or suicidal ideation/attempt (79.5%), sharp decrease in interest or pleasure (75.0%), and fatigue or loss of energy (70.5%). In contrast, only 20.5% of caregivers with depression experienced excessive or inappropriate feelings of guilt or inadequacy, the symptom least frequently mentioned.

Table 4. Depressive symptoms in caregivers with depression (*n* = 44)

Symptoms	Yes		No	
	n	%	*n*	%
Depressed mood	37	84.1	7	15.9
Sharp decrease in interest or pleasure	33	75.0	11	25.0
Significant weight loss or gain	35	79.5	9	20.5
Insomnia or hypersomnia	41	93.2	3	6.8
Psychomotor slowing or agitation	35	79.5	9	20.5
Fatigue or loss of energy	31	70.5	13	29.5
Feelings of excessive or inappropriate uselessness or guilt	9	20.5	35	79.5
Decreased ability to think or concentrate, or indecision	41	93.2	3	6.8
Recurrent thoughts of death, recurrent suicidal ideation, or suicide attempt or a specific plan to commit suicide	35	79.5	9	20.5

Variables Related to Depression

Table 5 shows the exploratory results of the univariate logistic regression analyses for major depressive disorder.

The variables found as potential predictors ($p \leq .30$) of depression were age, marital status, social class, employment situation, cause of dependence, burden, social support, and self-esteem.

Table 6 shows the predictors of major depressive disorder in the multivariate logistic regression analysis.

Table 5. Exploratory analyses: Results of bivariate logistic regression analyses for major depressive disorder

Potential predictor	OR (95% CI)	p
Age		
≤ 55 years	1.84 (0.96-3.54)	.067
> 55 years	1(ref)	
Marital status		
Single	1.69 (0.73-3.92)	.219
Partnered	1(ref)	
Social class		
Lower/Lower middle	0.69 (0.37-1.30)	.254
Upper middle/Upper	1(ref)	
Education		
No schooling/primary school	1.50 (0.57-3.94)	.415
Secondary education/university	1 (ref)	
Area of residence		
Rural	0.90 (0.48-1.67)	.731
Urban	1 (ref)	
Employment situation		
Employed	0.36 (0.11-1.18)	.091
High self-esteem (SES> 29)	1 (ref)	
Monthly household income		
< 1000 euros	0.88 (0.42-1.85)	.740
≥ 1000 euros	1 (ref)	
Sex of the care recipient		
Male	1.28 (0.65-2.50)	.473
Female	1 (ref)	
Age of the care recipient		
≤ 83	1.13 (0.61-2.10)	.704
> 83	1 (ref)	
Relationship with the caregiver		
Caring for a parent	1.09 (0.58-2.04)	.786
Caring for another person	1 (ref)	
Cause of dependence		
Dementia	1.72 (0.87-3.38)	.118
Other diseases	1 (ref)	
Duration of care (years)		
≤ 8 years	1.13 (0.61-2.10)	.704
> 8 years	1 (ref)	
Intensity of care (daily hours)		
≤ 12 hours	0.60 (0.21-1.73)	.342
> 12 hours	1 (ref)	
Burden		
Burdened (CBI > 24)	5.72 (2.49-13.14)	
Not burdened (CBI ≤ 24)	1 (ref)	<.001
Social support		
Low social support (Duke UNC < 32)	4.70 (2.47-8.94)	<.001
Normal social support (Duke UNC ≥ 32)	1 (ref)	
Self-esteem		
Low self-esteem (SES ≤ 29)	4.25 (2.23-8.09)	<.001

Table 6. Results of multivariate logistic regression analyses for major depressive disorder

Potential predictor	OR (95% CI)	*p*
Age		
≤ 55 years	1.52 (0.74-3.14)	.254
> 55 years	1(ref)	
Marital status		
Single	0.63 (0.26-1.53)	.304
Partnered	1(ref)	
Social class		
Lower/Lower middle	0.99 (0.48-2.01)	.970
Upper middle/Upper	1(ref)	
Employment situation		
Employed	0.40 (0.11-1.42)	.156
Unemployed	1 (ref)	
Cause of dependence		
Dementia	0.59 (0.28-1.22)	.154
Other diseases	1 (ref)	
Burden		
Burdened (CBI > 24)	3.87 (1.62-9.25)	.002
Not burdened (CBI ≤ 24)	1 (ref)	
Social support		
Low social support (Duke UNC < 32)	2.94 (1.45-5.98)	.003
Normal social support (Duke UNC ≥ 32)	1 (ref)	
Self-esteem		
Low self-esteem (SES ≤ 29)	2.85 (1.42-5.73)	.003
High self-esteem (SES> 29)	1 (ref)	

The variables that were predictive of major depressive disorder were being burdened (OR = 3.87, 95% CI, 1.62-9.25, $p = .002$), having low social support (OR = 2.94, 95% CI, 1.45-5.98, $p = .003$), and having low self-esteem (OR = 2.85, 95% CI, 1.42-5.73, $p = .003$).

DISCUSSION

One of the objectives of this study was to determine the sociodemographic profile of the care situation and clinical status in a representative sample of informal caregivers in Galicia. The 448 informal caregivers who participated in the study exhibited characteristics very similar to those found in previous studies. For example, informal caregivers' mean age of 54.2 years in this study aligns with that obtained in the work of Colombo et al. (2011), who describes a profile of informal caregivers over 45 years. Likewise, it is within the range found in the NAC and AARP report from 2009 (between 50 and 64 years old) or the study by García-Calvente et al. (2011; between 45 and 64 years old). The average age in the present study was slightly below the range found in the work of Spillman et al. 2014 (between 55 and 64 years) and Pickard's (2011) study, where most of the caregivers were more than 65 years old.

Our data on the marital status of caregivers are consistent with those previously found in other investigations, which report that most caregivers are married or living as a couple. In the present study, 76.6% of caregivers were women, compared to 71.3% found by García-Calvente et al. (2011) and 59% from the NAC and AARP 2009 report. Pickard´s (2011) study found most caregivers were married, consistently with our findings.

In relation to the educational level of the caregivers, this study found that 84.4% of participants had not attended school or had only completed primary education. Likewise, this figure is in line with the findings of some previous research, which agrees in pointing out that the educational level of caregivers is low. This is indicated in the work of Pickard (2011), where 63% of caregivers had a primary education, the work of García-Calvente et al. (2011), and the 76% figure found in Martínez, López, & Cuéllar (2013). In this study, 15.6% of caregivers had a secondary or tertiary educational level, lower than the one found in the NAC and AARP (2009) study, where 26% of caregivers had attended university.

Regarding the area of residence, 52.5% of caregivers lived in rural areas. This figure contrasts with that obtained in the NAC and AARP (2009) study, where 39% of caregivers resided in suburban areas and 29% in urban areas, with caregivers in rural areas representing a minority (around 31%).

In relation to work situation, this study found only 16.1% of caregivers had a paid job, a finding similar to that of García-Calvente et al. (2011) and by Martínez et al. (2013), in which 25.5% and 23.3% of caregivers were employed, respectively. However, the data contrast with what was found in the work of NAC and AARP, where 61% of caregivers had a paid job, and

Colombo et al. (2011), where this percentage was somewhat lower than 60% for the countries of southern Europe.

Regarding the care recipient, the data obtained in this study are consistent with those found in the NAC and AARP (2009) study. Most of the dependent persons were women (68%, according to the NAC and AARP (2009) study, and 72.8% in this study) and are at an advanced age (more than 75 years old, according to the NAC and AARP (2009) study and of an average of 74.2 years in this investigation).

Regarding the kinship relationship that unites the informal caregiver with the care recipient, the findings reveal that in most cases the caregiver is the daughter, with percentages ranging between 29.3% and 64% (Hoffmann & Rodrigues, 2010; Martínez et al. 2013; NAC and AARP 2009; Spillman et al. 2014). The data obtained in this study also point in this direction, with 43.5% of caregivers taking care of a parent.

In relation to the cause of dependence, 40.6% of caregivers from our study cared for people suffering from dementia. These figures are higher but in line with the data from the work of Spillman et al. (2014), where 33% of caregivers cared for persons with probable dementia, and with the NAC and AARP (2009) report, where 15% of situations were associated with dependence caused by advanced age, and an additional 15% with Alzheimer's or memory loss.

There is less consensus among the studies regarding the duration and intensity of care. The present sample found that the participants spent an average of 11.4 years providing care and devoted an average of 16.6 hours per day to this work. These data are close to what was reported by García-Calvente et al. (2011; more than 8 years of care, with a very high intensity of more than 15 hours a day), and data on the intensity of care reported by Crespo and López (2007; 101.9 hours of care per week, equivalent to about 14.6 hours of care per day); however, they are higher than the figures found in other studies for duration of care (an average duration of 5.8 years in the work of Crespo and López [2007] and 1–4 years in the NAC and AARP [2009] report) and for intensity of care (1–8 hours per day in the NAC and AARP [2009] report, around 50 hours per week in Hoffmann and Rodrigues [2010], equivalent to 7.1 hours per day; between 10 and 20 hours per week in the study by Colombo et al. [2011], equivalent to between 1.4 and 2.9 hours per day; or 75.1 hours per month from Spillman et al. [2014], equivalent to around 2.5 hours a day).

In relation to the clinical variables, 51.6% of caregivers in this study were burdened. This percentage was more than double that found in a previous work carried out in Singapore with persons providing care for elderly people (Vaingankar et al. 2016), which used the same evaluation instrument and a similar cutoff point, finding 24.5% of caregivers to be burdened.

Regarding social support, 27.0% of caregivers had low social support and 73.0% had normal social support; this data is similar to those found in the works of Quinn, Briggs, Miller, & Orellana (2014), where 23.7% of caregivers reported having little social support; and Del Río-Lozano, García-Calvente, Calle-Romero, Machón-Sobrado, & Larrañaga-Padilla (2017), where 78.0% of caregivers reported having high social support.

Regarding self-esteem, 30.6% of caregivers in this study had low self-esteem and 69.4% had high self-esteem. Although there are no previous studies that have analyzed the prevalence of low self-esteem in caregivers, this figure is more positive than the percentage found in previous studies in other populations, such as community mental health nurses (Fothergill, Edwards, Hannigan, Burnard, & Coyle, 2000), who reported low self-esteem in 40% of cases. This finding, which might seem contradictory, is supported by previous research that indicates that some caregivers obtain subjective benefits from the role they play, which include a sense of personal growth and usefulness, satisfaction from being close to the person they care for, and pride in one's ability to handle critical situations (Kramer, 1997; Ott, Sanders & Kelber, 2007).

On the other hand, a second objective of this project was to determine the prevalence of major depressive episodes in the caregivers comprising the selected sample, finding a prevalence of 9.8%. This figure is higher than the one found for women in the Spanish general population, which ranges from a one-month prevalence of 2.6% (Ayuso-Mateos et al., 2001) to a 12-month prevalence of 5.7% (Gabilondo et al. 2010). However, in estimates from samples of informal caregivers, the data obtained in this study contrast with those found in previous national and international studies, with percentages ranging between 14% and 55% (Cohen et al., 1990; Gallagher et al., 1989; Grunfeld et al., 2004; Redinbaugh, et al., 1995; Schulz et al., 1995). The most plausible explanation for this discrepancy is that these studies, unlike ours, were conducted using convenience samples and did not use explicit diagnostic criteria, such as those included in the Diagnostic and Statistical Manual of Mental Disorders (DSM) or the International Classification of Diseases (ICD).

The depressive symptoms most frequently observed in the caregivers from the present study are insomnia (93.2%), decreased ability to think or concentrate (93.2%), and depressed mood (84.1%). These findings differ from those found in the general population, among whom the most frequent symptoms for people with depression are insomnia, fatigue, and recurrent thoughts of death (Judd, Rapaport, Paulus, & Brown, 1994). Caregivers frequently experience sleep disturbances, with and without major depression, which are presumably linked to nocturnal behaviors of the care recipient (Creese, Bédard, Brazil, & Chambers, 2008). However, the percentages, and in particular the ones related to sleep disorders, were higher than those found in previous studies of informal caregivers (e.g., McCurry, Logsdon, Teri, & Vitiello, 2007).

The third and final objective of this study was to examine the relationship between major depressive episodes and different variables of the caregiver, the care recipient, the care situation, and the caregiver's clinical characteristics. According to data found in the present study, none of the variables analyzed regarding the sociodemographic profile of the caregiver, the care recipient, or the care situation was significantly related to depression. These results are in line with previous findings, there being no difference found in terms of the type of tie between the caregiver and the care recipient (Crespo & López, 2007), and in relation to the disorder causing dependence (Crespo et al., 2005). However, the other variables disagree with previous research. For example, different studies suggest that age is a significant predictor of depression, and as such younger caregivers would be more vulnerable (Blanco et al., 2014; Covinsky et al., 2003; Crespo & López, 2007). There is also a certain consensus in indicating that family income is associated with depression, with low-income caregivers at a higher risk of experiencing a depressive episode (Crespo & López, 2007; Majerovitz, 2007; Wang et al., 2016; Williams et al., 2003). Also, different studies coincide in finding that low educational level increases the risk of developing depression (Covinsky et al., 2003; Crespo & López, 2007; Lee et al., 2015; Lu et al., 2007). Other research has linked depression with being single (Derajew et al., 2017), member of the upper class (Blanco et al., 2014), resident in urban areas (Bigbee et al., 2011; Imaiso et al., 2012; Lee et al., 2010), and unemployed (Lee et al., 2015). In relation to the variables concerning the care situation, previous research has linked depression in caregivers with caring for a younger male (Covinsky et al., 2003; Pinquart & Sörensen, 2011; Chappell et al., 2015). However, once again, the differences in the instruments used to establish depression—diagnostic interview versus the use of self-report scales of depressive symptoms—limit the comparison.

In relation to the clinical variables, level of burden, social support, and self-esteem were all predictors of depression. It was found that caregivers who were burdened were more likely to suffer clinical depression (adjusted OR = 3.87, 95% CI [1.62- 9.25]). These data are consistent with the results of earlier studies that found a relationship between caregiver burden and an increase in the likelihood of caregivers developing depressive symptoms or even experiencing an episode of major depression (Epstein-Lubow et al., 2008; Gallagher et al., 2008; Grunfeld et al., 2004; Li, 2005; O'Rourke, & Tuokko, 2004; Perlick et al., 2016; Tsai & Pai, 2016). Regarding social support, caregivers with low perceived social support were at a higher risk of depression (adjusted OR = 2.94, 95% CI [1.45-5.98]) than those who perceived themselves to have a normal level of social support. These data provide additional empirical support for the results of several studies that have found that social support plays a protective role against depression in caregivers (Ali & Kausar, 2016; Brummett et al. 2012; Majerovitz 2007; Pagel & Becker, 1987). One of these studies was specifically conducted with female caregivers (Casale et al., 2015). Finally, self-esteem also acted as a protective factor against depression in this population; caregivers with low self-esteem were more likely to be depressed than those with high self-esteem (adjusted OR = 2.85, 95% CI [1.42-5.73]). This finding is consistent with previous studies that have found low self-esteem predicting depressive symptoms in the caregiver population, while high self-esteem reduces the risk of depression in the same population (Chung et al., 2016; Land et al., 2003; Pagel & Becker, 1987; Zunzunegui et al., 2002).

This study has several strengths. First, it was carried out using face-to-face clinical interviews, which allows the research instruments to be administered correctly and avoids bias due to missing or incomplete answers (Weinberger, Oddone, Samsa, & Landsman, 1996). In addition, it used a randomized representative sample of caregivers for people suffering from all types of disorders that give rise to dependence. Caregivers experiencing episodes of major depression were identified by trained interviewers using the SCID-CV as an aid in establishing this diagnosis.

However, this study also has some limitations. First, it employs a cross-sectional design, and it could only evaluate associations but not causal relationships. A cross-sectional design is not able to capture differences in informal caregivers' depression across time or in response to the changing clinical condition of the care recipient (Grunfeld et al., 2004). In addition, the diagnostic interview did not evaluate psychiatric comorbidity, which creates some uncertainty about the strength of the correlations and the specificity of the variables associated with depression contrasted with psychiatric disorders in general. The study did not evaluate the quality of care provided by caregivers, and so we cannot reach conclusions on whether informal caregivers currently experiencing major depression provide lower-quality care than those without depression, as Williamson & Shaffer (2001) indicate, although this is certainly plausible.

This study has important implications for policy, clinical practice, and the provision of services. Properly documenting the prevalence of depression in the informal caregiver population is essential for governments, medical centers, and social services, as it provides the necessary information to estimate the need for adequate preventive and treatment services and interventions to support this population. Given the high prevalence of depression this study found in informal caregivers compared to the general population and given that depression significantly impairs functioning and may compromise caregivers' ability to care for others, clinicians should be vigilant to its evaluation and diagnosis. If depressive symptoms are simply considered a normal response to the stressful situation of caring for someone with a long-term illness or disability, this may lead to a failure to detect, prevent, and treat depressive disorders among caregivers. On the other hand, we must not forget that it has been documented that depression in caregivers is associated with a low quality of life, premature institutionalization, and mistreatment of the care recipient (Karlawish, Casarett, Klocinski, & Clark, 2001).

Finally, it should be noted that future studies, in addition to evaluating comorbidity, might find it useful to use self-report scales that could add supplemental information on the severity of depressive symptoms. However, it is important to bear in mind that the objective of this study was to determine the prevalence of episodes of major depression, and it employed the current standard procedure considered the most appropriate to establishing such a diagnosis in a research context. Given the results obtained, it would be useful to make such evaluations taking gender into consideration and to address specific aspects that particularly affect women who provide care for their dependent relatives. This would facilitate the design of programs to prevent and treat depression targeted especially at this population (e.g., Otero et al., 2015; Vázquez et al., 2016). Likewise, when considering the treatment options that informal caregivers need, future studies could include other instruments to assess the quality of care they provide and consider certain important subjective perceptions of informal caregivers.

In conclusion, our finding that episodes of major depression are quite prevalent among informal caregivers for dependent persons, regardless of their sociodemographic profile, suggests that an important goal of health care policy is to ensure psychological and psychiatric follow-up to guarantee their mental health and well-being. Likewise, the findings that burden constitutes a risk factor for depression, while social support and self-esteem are protective factors, provide relevant information for the development of clinical interventions targeting this population.

CONCLUSION

The following conclusions can be established considering this study's results:

1. The most common characteristics of informal caregivers in this study were that they were middle-aged women, married or living with a partner, middle class, with only a primary education, residing in a rural environment, whose main activity is housework and a monthly household income of 1000 euros or more, handling care for their parents. The time they devote to this role is significant and continuous: approximately 16 hours a day for more than 11 years.
2. The most common characteristics of the care recipient were that they were elderly women, a parent of the informal caregiver, and dependent as a result of dementia.
3. In relation to the clinical profile of caregivers, they tended to have a high level of burden, normal social support, and high self-esteem compared to non-caregiver populations.
4. Of the total of 448 informal caregivers who participated in this study, 9.8% were experiencing an episode of major depression at the present time according to DSM criteria.
5. The most frequent depressive symptoms that caregivers experienced were, in order: insomnia, decreased ability to think or concentrate, and depressive mood.
6. There were no significant differences between caregivers with and without depression with respect to age, marital status, social class, educational level, area of residence, employment status, monthly income, sex of the care recipient, age of the care recipient, relationship of the care recipient with the caregiver, cause of dependence, duration of care, or intensity of care
7. Experiencing burden and having low social support and low self-esteem were associated with an increased risk of depression.
8. The high prevalence of depression found here should help to raise awareness of the urgent need for prevention and treatment programs

aimed at this population. Future studies could include other assessment instruments in order to obtain information that supplements the aspects evaluated in this study, such as the severity of depressive symptoms, psychiatric comorbidities, or quality of care provided by caregivers. It would be advisable to introduce a gender perspective in these evaluations, addressing specific aspects that affect the group of informal caregivers.

References

Ali, N., & Kausar, R. (2016). Social support and coping as predictors of psychological distress in family caregivers of stroke patients. *Pakistan Journal of Psychological Research, 31*(2), 587-608.

Argyriou, A. A., Karanasios, P., Ifanti, A. A., Iconomou, G., Assimakopoulos, K., Makridou, A., ... Makris, N. (2011). Quality of life and emotional burden of primary caregivers: A case–control study of multiple sclerosis patients in Greece. *Quality of Life Research: An International Journal of Quality of Life Aspects of Treatment, Care & Rehabilitation, 20*(10), 1663-1668. doi: 10.1007/s11136-011-9899-2

Austen, S., & Ong, R. (2013). The effects of ill health and informal care roles on the employment retention of mid-life women: Does the workplace matter? *Journal of Industrial Relations, 55*, 663–680. doi: 10.1177/0022185613494648.

Ayuso-Mateos, J., Vázquez-Barquero, J. L., Dowrick, C., Lehtinen, V., Dalgard, O. S., Casey, P., ... Wilkinson, G. (2001). Depressive disorders in Europe: Prevalence figures from the ODIN study. *The British Journal of Psychiatry, 179*(4), 308-316. doi:10.1192/bjp.179.4.308.

Baillie, V., Norbeck, J. S., & Barnes, L. E. (1988). Stress, social support, and psychological distress of family caregivers of the elderly. *Nursing Research, 37*(4), 217-222. doi: 10.1097/00006199-198807000-00009.

Bellón, J. A., Delgado, A., Luna del Castillo, J. D., & Lardelli, P. (1996). [Validity and reliability of the Duke-UNC-11 questionnaire of functional social support]. *Atencion Primaria, 18*(4), 153.

Bigbee, J. L., Musil, C., & Kenski, D. (2011). The health of caregiving grandmothers: A rural-urban comparison. *The Journal of Rural Health, 27*(3), 289-296. doi: 10.1111/j.1748-0361.2010.00340.x.

Blanco, V., Guisande, M. A., Sánchez, M. T., Otero, P., López, L., & Vázquez, F. L. (2019). Síndrome de carga del cuidador y factores asociados en cuidadores familiares gallegos [Caregiver burden syndrome and associated factors in Galician family caregivers]. *Revista Española De Geriatría y Gerontología, 54*(1), 19-26. doi: 10.1016/j.regg.2018.03.005.

Blanco, V., Rohde, P., Vázquez, F. L., & Torres, Á. (2014). Identification of caregivers at greatest risk of major depression in two prevention studies. *Psychotherapy Research, 24*(5), 578-593. doi: 10.1080/10503307.2013.847989.

Brislin, R. W., Lonner, W. J., & Thorndike, R. M. (1973). *Cross-cultural research methods*. New York: Wiley.

Broadhead, W. E., Gehlbach, S. H., de Gruy, F. V., & Kaplan, B. H. (1988). The Duke–UNC functional social support questionnaire: Measurement of social support in family medicine patients. *Medical Care, 26*(7), 709-723. doi: 10.1097/00005650-198807000-00006.

Brummett, B. H., Siegler, I. C., Williams, R. B., Hilliard, T. S., & Dilworth-Anderson, P. (2012). Associations of social support and 8-year follow-up depressive symptoms: Differences in African-American and White caregivers. *Clinical Gerontologist: The Journal of Aging and Mental Health, 35*(4), 289-302. doi: 10.1080/07317115.2012.678569.

Capistrant, B. D., Berkman, L. F., & Glymour, M. M. (2014). Does duration of spousal caregiving affect risk of depression onset? Evidence from the health and retirement study. *The American Journal of Geriatric Psychiatry, 22*(8), 766-770. doi: 10.1016/j.jagp.2013.01.073.

Casale, M., Wild, L., Cluver, L., & Kuo, C. (2015). Social support as a protective factor for depression among women caring for children in HIV-endemic South Africa. *Journal of Behavioral Medicine, 38*(1), 17-27. doi: 10.1007/s10865-014-9556-7.

Chappell, N. L., Dujela, C., & Smith, A. (2015). Caregiver well-being: Intersections of relationship and gender. *Research on Aging, 37*(6), 623-645. doi: 10.1177/0164027514549258.

Chung, M. L., Bakas, T., Plue, L. D., & Williams, L. S. (2016). Effects of self-esteem, optimism, and perceived control on depressive symptoms in stroke survivor-spouse dyads. *Journal of Cardiovascular Nursing, 31*(2), E8-E16. doi: 10.1097/JCN.0000000000000232.

Cohen, D., Luchins, D., Eisdorfer, C., Paveza, G. J., Ashford, J. W., Gorelick, P.,...Shaw, H. (1990). Caring for relatives with Alzheimer's disease: The mental health risks to spouses, adult children, and other family caregivers. *Behavior, Health, & Aging, 1*(3), 171-182.

Colombo, F., Llena-Nozal, A., Mercier, J., & Tjadens, F. (2011). *Help wanted? Providing and paying for long-term care.* Paris: OECD Publishing. Retrieved from: https://ec.europa.eu/health/sites/health/files/state/docs/oecd_helpwanted _en.pdf.

Covinsky, K. E., Newcomer, R., Fox, P., Wood, J., Sands, L., Dane, K., & Yaffe, K. (2003). Patient and caregiver characteristics associated with depression in caregivers of patients with dementia. *Journal of General Internal Medicine, 18*(12), 1006-1014. doi: 10.1111/j.1525-1497.2003.30103.x.

Creese, J., Bédard, M., Brazil, K., & Chambers, L. (2008). Sleep disturbances in spousal caregivers of individuals with Alzheimer's disease. *International Psychogeriatrics, 20*(1), 149-161. doi: 10.1017/S1041610207005339.

Crespo, M., & López, J. (2007). *El apoyo a los cuidadores de familiares mayores dependientes en el hogar: desarrollo del programa "Cómo mantener su* bienestar" [Support to caregivers of the family elderly at home: development of the program "How to preserve your well-being"]. Madrid: Ministerio de Trabajo y Asuntos Sociales. Retrieved from: http://www.imserso.es/InterPresent1/groups/imserso/documents/binario/apoyocuidadores.pdf.

Crespo, M., López, J., & Zarit, S. H. (2005). Depression and anxiety in primary caregivers: A comparative study of caregivers of demented and nondemented older persons. *International Journal of Geriatric Psychiatry, 20*(6), 591-592. doi: 10.1002/gps.1321.

Cuijpers, P. (2005). Depressive disorders in caregivers of dementia patients: A systematic review. *Aging & Mental Health, 9*(4), 325-330. doi: 10.1080/13607860500090078.

Del Pino, R., Frías, A., Palomino, P. A., & Martínez-Riera, J. R. (2012). Gender differences regarding informal caregivers of older people. *Journal of Nursing Scholarship, 44*(4), 349-357. doi:10.1111/j.1547-5069.2012.01477.x.

Del Río-Lozano, M., García-Calvente, M. M., Calle-Romero, J., Machón-Sobrado, M., & Larrañaga-Padilla, I. (2017). Health-related quality of life in Spanish informal caregivers: Gender differences and support received. *Quality of Life Research: An International Journal of Quality of Life Aspects of Treatment, Care & Rehabilitation, 26*(12), 3227-3238. doi: 10.1007/s11136-017-1678-2.

Dentinger, E., & Clarkberg, M. (2002). Informal caregiving and retirement timing among men and women: Gender and caregiving relationships in late midlife. *Journal of Family Issues, 23*(7), 857-879. doi: 10.1177/019251302236598.

Derajew, H., Tolessa, D., Feyissa, G. T., Addisu, F., & Soboka, M. (2017). Prevalence of depression and its associated factors among primary caregivers of patients with severe mental illness in Southwest Ethiopia. *BMC Psychiatry, 17*, 8. doi: 10.1186/s12888-017-1249-7.

Epstein-Lubow, G., Davis, J. D., Miller, I. W., & Tremont, G. (2008). Persisting burden predicts depressive symptoms in dementia caregivers. *Journal of Geriatric Psychiatry and Neurology, 21*(3), 198-203. doi: 10.1177/0891988708320972.

Feinberg, L., & Pilisuk. T. (1999). *Survey of Fifteen States Caregiver Support Programs: Final Report*. San Francisco: Family Caregiver Alliance.

Fernández-Montalvo, J., & Echeburúa, E. (1997). Variables psicopatológicas y distorsiones cognitivas de los maltratadores en el hogar: Un análisis descriptivo [Psychopathological variables and cognitive distortions of abusers at home: A descriptive analysis]. *Análisis y Modificación De Conducta, 23*(88), 151-180.

First, M. B., Spitzer, R. L., Gibbon, M., & Williams, J. B. W. (1999). *Entrevista clínica estructurada para los trastornos del Eje I del DSM-IV-Versión clínica (SCID-CV)* [*Structured clinical interview for DSM-IV Axis I disorders—Clinical version (SCID-CV)*]. Barcelona: Masson.

First, M. B., Spitzer, R. L., Gibbon, M., & Williams, J. B. W. (2000). *User´s guide for the Structured Clinical Interview for DSM-IV Axis I Disorders-Clinician Version (SCID-CV).* Washington DC: American Psychiatric Press.

Fothergill, A., Edwards, D., Hannigan, B., Burnard, P., & Coyle, D. (2000). Self-esteem in community mental health nurses: Findings from the all-Wales stress study. *Journal of Psychiatric and Mental Health Nursing, 7*(4), 315-321. doi: 10.1046/j.1365-2850.2000.00323.x.

Gabilondo, A., Rojas-Farreras, S., Vilagut, G., Haro, J. M., Fernández, A., Pinto-Meza, A., & Alonso, J. (2010). Epidemiology of major depressive episode in a southern European country: Results from the ESEMeD-spain project. *Journal of Affective Disorders, 120*(1-3), 76-85. doi: 10.1016/j.jad.2009.04.016.

Gallagher, D., Rose, J., Rivera, P., Lovett, S., & Thompson, L. W. (1989). Prevalence of depression in family caregivers. *The Gerontologist, 29*(4), 449-456. doi: 10.1093/geront/29.4.449.

Gallagher, S., Phillips, A. C., Oliver, C., & Carroll, D. (2008). Predictors of psychological morbidity in parents of children with intellectual disabilities. *Journal of Pediatric Psychology, 33*(10), 1129-1136. doi: 10.1093/jpepsy/jsn040.

García-Calvente, M. M., Mateo-Rodríguez, I., & Eguiguren, A. P. (2004). [The system of informal caregiving as inequality]. *Gaceta Sanitaria, 18 Suppl 1*, 132–139.

García-Calvente, M. M., Mateo-Rodríguez, I., & Maroto-Navarro, G. (2004). [Impact of caregiving on women's health and quality of life]. *Gaceta Sanitaria, 18 Suppl 2*, 83–92.

García-Calvente, M., Del Río, M., & Marcos, J. (2011). [Gender inequalities in health deterioration as a result of informal care in Spain]. *Gaceta Sanitaria, 25 Suppl 2*, 100–107. doi: 10.1016/j.gaceta.2011.09.006.

Grunfeld, E., Coyle, D., Whelan, T., Clinch, J., Reyno, L., Earle, C. C., .. Glossop, R. (2004). Family caregiver burden: Results of a longitudinal study of breast cancer patients and their principal caregivers. *Canadian Medical Association Journal, 170*(12), 1795-1801. doi: 10.1503/cmaj.1031205.

Guerriere, D., Husain, A., Zagorski, B., Marshall, D., Seow, H., Brazil, K., ... Coyte, P. C. (2016). Predictors of caregiver burden across the home-based palliative care trajectory in Ontario, Canada. *Health & Social Care in the Community, 24*(4), 428-438. doi: 10.1111/hsc.12219.

Guillemin, F., Bombardier, C., & Beaton, D. (1993). Cross-cultural adaptation of health-related quality of life measures: Literature review and proposed guidelines. *Journal of Clinical Epidemiology, 46*(12), 1417-1432. doi: 10.1016/0895-4356(93)90142-N.

Hammond, T., Weinberg, M. K., & Cummins, R. A. (2014). The dyadic interaction of relationships and disability type on informal carer subjective well-being. *Quality of Life Research: An International Journal of Quality of Life Aspects of Treatment, Care & Rehabilitation, 23*(5), 1535-1542. doi: 10.1007/s11136-013-0577-4.

Harwood, R. H., Sayer, A. A., & Hirschfeld, M. (2004). Current and future worldwide prevalence of dependency, its relationship to total population, and dependency ratios. *Bulletin of the World Health Organization*, *82*(4), 251–258.

Hoffmann, F., & Rodrigues, R. (2010). *Informal carers: Who takes care of them? Policy Brief April 2010*. Vienna: European Centre for Social Welfare Policy and Research. Retrieved from: https://www.euro.centre.org/downloads/detail/1256.

Imaiso, J., Tsukasaki, K., & Okoshi, F. (2012). Differences in home-based family caregiving appraisal for caregivers of the elderly in rural and urban Japanese communities. *Journal of Community Health Nursing, 29*(1), 25-38. doi: 10.1080/07370016.2012.645733.

Jácome, C., Figueiredo, D., Gabriel, R., Cruz, J., & Marques, A. (2014). Predicting anxiety and depression among family carers of people with chronic obstructive pulmonary disease. *International Psychogeriatrics, 26*(7), 1191-1199. doi: 10.1017/S1041610214000337.

Jamieson, A. (1993). Atención informal en Europa [Informal care in Europe]. In A. Jamieson, & R. Illsley (Ed.), *Comparación de políticas Europeas de Atención a Personas Ancianas* [Comparison of European eldercare policies]. (pp.13-32). Barcelona: SG editores.

Jenson, J., & Jacobzone, S. (2000). *Care allowances for the frail elderly and their impact on women caregivers. Labour Market and Social Policy – Occasional Papers nº 41. Paris: OECD.*

Joling, K. J., Smit, F., van Marwijk, H. W. J., van der Host, H. E., Scheltens, P., Schulz, R., & van Hout, H. P. J. (2012). Identifying target groups for the prevention of depression among caregivers of dementia patients. *International Psychogeriatrics, 24*(2), 298-306. doi: 10.1017/S1041610211001633.

Joling, K. J., van Hout, H. P. J., Schellevis, F. G., van der Host, H. E., Scheltens, P., Knol, D. L., & van Marwijk, H. W. J. (2010). Incidence of depression and anxiety in the spouses of patients with dementia: A naturalistic cohort study of recorded morbidity with a 6-year follow-up. *The American Journal of Geriatric Psychiatry, 18*(2), 146-153. doi: 10.1097/JGP.0b013e3181bf9f0f.

Judd, L. L., Rapaport, M. H., Paulus, M. P., & Brown, J. L. (1994). Subsyndromal symptomatic depression: A new mood disorder? *The Journal of Clinical Psychiatry, 55*(4), 18-28.

Karlawish, J. H., Casarett, D., Klocinski, J., & Clark, C. M. (2001). The relationship between caregivers' global ratings of Alzheimer's disease patients' quality of life, disease severity, and the caregiving experience. *Journal of the American Geriatrics Society*, *49*(8), 1066–1070.

Kim, Y., & Schulz, R. (2008). Family caregivers' strains: Comparative analysis of cancer caregiving with dementia, diabetes, and frail elderly caregiving. *Journal of Aging and Health, 20*(5), 483-503. doi: 10.1177/0898264308317533.

Kim, Y., Shaffer, K. M., Carver, C. S., & Cannady, R. S. (2014). Prevalence and predictors of depressive symptoms among cancer caregivers 5 years after the relative's cancer diagnosis. *Journal of Consulting and Clinical Psychology, 82*(1), 1-8. doi: 10.1037/a0035116.

Koyama, A., Matsushita, M., Hashimoto, M., Fujise, N., Ishikawa, T., Tanaka, H., ... Ikeda, M. (2017). Mental health among younger and older caregivers of dementia patients. *Psychogeriatrics, 17*(2), 108-114. doi: 10.1111/psyg.12200.

Kramer, B. J. (1997). Gain in the caregiving experience: Where are we? What next? *The Gerontologist, 37*(2), 218-232. doi: 10.1093/geront/ 37.2.218.

Kuscu, M. K., Dural, U., Önen, P., Yaşa, Y., Yayla, M., Basaran, G., ... Bekiroğlu, N. (2009). The association between individual attachment patterns, the perceived social support, and the psychological well-being of Turkish informal caregivers. *Psycho-Oncology, 18*(9), 927-935. doi: 10.1002/pon.v18:910.1002/pon.1441.

Land, H., Hudson, S. M., & Stiefel, B. (2003). Stress and depression among HIV-positive and HIV-negative gay and bisexual AIDS caregivers. *AIDS and Behavior, 7*(1), 41-53. doi: 10.1023/A:1022509306761.

Lee, Y., Lin, P., Chien, C., & Fang, F. (2015). Prevalence and risk factors of depressive disorder in caregivers of patients with head and neck cancer. *Psycho-Oncology, 24*(2), 155-161. doi: 10.1002/pon.3619.

Lee, Y., & Tang, F. (2015). More caregiving, less working: Caregiving roles and gender difference. *Journal of Applied Gerontology, 34*(4), 465-483. doi: 10.1177/0733464813508649.

Lee, J., Yoo, M. S., & Jung, D. (2010). Caregiving appraisal of family caregivers for older stroke patients in Korea. *International Nursing Review, 57*(1), 107-112. doi: 10.1111/j.1466-7657.2009.00751.x.

Li, L. W. (2005). From caregiving to bereavement: Trajectories of depressive symptoms among wife and daughter caregivers. *The Journals of Gerontology: Series B: Psychological Sciences and Social Sciences, 60*(4), P190-P198. doi: 10.1093/geronb/60.4.P190.

Livingston, G., Manela, M., & Katona, C. (1996). Depression and Other Psychiatric Morbidity in Carers of Elderly People Living at Home.

British Medical Journal (Clinical Research Ed.), 312, 153-156. doi: 10.1136/bmj.312.7024.153.

Lu, Y. Y., Austrom, M. G., Perkins, S. M., Bakas, T., Farlow, M. R., He, F.,... Gamst, A. (2007). Depressed mood in informal caregivers of individuals with mild cognitive impairment. *American Journal of Alzheimer's Disease and Other Dementias, 22*(4), 273-285. doi: 10.1177/1533317507301367.

Mahoney, R., Regan, C., Katona, C., & Livingston, G. (2005). Anxiety and depression in family caregivers of people with Alzheimer disease: The LASER-AD study. *The American Journal of Geriatric Psychiatry, 13*(9), 795-801. doi: 10.1176/appi.ajgp.13.9.795.

Majerovitz, S. D. (2007). Predictors of burden and depression among nursing home family caregivers. *Aging & Mental Health, 11*(3), 323-329. doi: 10.1080/13607860600963380.

Martínez, M. E., López, M. P., & Cuéllar, I. (2013). Salud y sobrecarga percibida en personas cuidadoras familiares de una zona rural [Health and perceived burden in caregivers from a rural area]. *Clínica y Salud, 24*(1), 37-45. doi:10.5093/cl2013a5.

Masanet, E., & La Parra, D. (2011). Relationship between the number of hours of informal care and the mental health status of caregivers. *Revista Española De Salud Pública, 85* (3) (06), 257–266. doi: 10.1590/S1135-57272011000300004.

McCurry, S. M., Logsdon, R. G., Teri, L., & Vitiello, M. V. (2007). Sleep disturbances in caregivers of persons with dementia: Contributing factors and treatment implications. *Sleep Medicine Reviews, 11*(2), 143-153. doi: 10.1016/j.smrv.2006.09.002.

Mittelman, M. S., Roth, D. I., Clay, O. J., & Haley, W. E. (2007). Preserving health of Alzheimer's caregivers: Impact of a spouse caregiver intervention. *The American Journal of Geriatric Psychiatry, 15*(9), 780-789. doi: 10.1097/JGP.0b013e31805d858a.

Morgan, T., Williams, L. A., Trussardi, G., & Gott, M. (2016). Gender and family caregiving at the end-of-life in the context of old age: A systematic review. *Palliative Medicine, 30*(7), 616-624. doi: 10.1177/0269216315625857.

Muller, C., & Volkov, O. (2009). Older women: Work and caregiving in conflict? A study of four countries. *Social Work in Health Care, 48*(7), 665-695. doi: 10.1080/00981380902921732.

National Alliance for Caregiving [NAC] and AARP. (2009). *Caregiving in the US. 2009*. Retrieved from: http://www.caregiving.org/data/FINAL Regular ExSum50plus.pdf.

Neary, M. A. (1993). Type of elder impairment: Impact on caregiver burden, health outcomes and social support. *Clinical Gerontologist: The Journal of Aging and Mental Health, 13*(2), 47-59. doi: 10.1300/J018v13n02_04.

Newman, T. B., Browner, W. S., Cummings, S. R., & Hulley, S. B. (2008). Diseño de estudios transversales y de casos y controles [Design of cross-sectional studies, case studies, and control studies]. In S. B. Hulley, S. R. Cummings, W. S. Browner, D. G. Grady, & T. B. Newman (Eds.), *Diseño de investigaciones clínicas* [Design of clinical research], 4th ed. (pp. 121-141). Barcelona: Wolters Kluwer.

O'Rourke, N., & Tuokko, H. A. (2004). Caregiver burden and depressive symptomatology: The association between constructs over time. *Clinical Gerontologist: The Journal of Aging and Mental Health, 27*(4), 41-52. doi: 10.1300/J018v27n04_05.

Otero, P., Smit, F., Cuijpers, P., Torres, A., Blanco, V., & Vázquez, F. L. (2015). Long-term efficacy of indicated prevention of depression in non-professional caregivers: Randomized controlled trial. *Psychological Medicine, 45*(7), 1401-1412. doi: 10.1017/S0033291714002505.

Ott, C. H., Sanders, S., & Kelber, S. T. (2007). Grief and personal growth experience of spouses and adult-child caregivers of individuals with Alzheimer's disease and related dementias. *The Gerontologist, 47*(6), 798-809. doi:http://dx.doi.org/10.1093/geront/47.6.798.

Pagel, M., & Becker, J. (1987). Depressive thinking and depression: Relations with personality and social resources. *Journal of Personality and Social Psychology, 52*(5), 1043-1052. doi: 10.1037/0022-3514.52.5.1043.

Perlick, D. A., Berk, L., Kaczynski, R., Gonzalez, J., Link, B., Dixon, L., ... Miklowitz, D. J. (2016). Caregiver burden as a predictor of depression among family and friends who provide care for persons with bipolar disorder. *Bipolar Disorders, 18*(2), 183-191. doi: 10.1111/bdi.12379.

Pickard, L. (2011). *The supply of informal care in Europe. ENEPRI Research Report No. 94.* Retrieved from: http://aei.pitt.edu/32514/1/ENEPRI_RR94__ANCIEN_WP_3__Supply_of_Informal_Care_in_Europe.pdf.

Pinquart, M., & Sörensen, S. (2003). Differences between caregivers and noncaregivers in psychological health and physical health: A meta-analysis. *Psychology and Aging, 18*(2), 250-267. doi: 10.1037/0882-7974.18.2.250.

Pinquart, M., & Sörensen, S. (2006). Gender differences in caregiver stressors, social resources, and health: An updated meta-analysis. *The Journals of Gerontology: Series B: Psychological Sciences and Social Sciences, 61*(1), P33-P45. doi: 10.1093/geronb/61.1.P33.

Pinquart, M., & Sörensen, S. (2007). Correlates of physical health of informal caregivers: A meta-analysis. *The Journals of Gerontology: Series B: Psychological Sciences and Social Sciences, 62*(2), P126-P137. doi: 10.1093/geronb/62.2.P126.

Pinquart, M., & Sörensen, S. (2011). Spouses, adult children, and children-in-law as caregivers of older adults: A meta-analytic comparison. *Psychology and Aging, 26*(1), 1-14. doi: 10.1037/a0021863.

Quinn, A., Briggs, H. E., Miller, K. M., & Orellana, E. R. (2014). Social and familial determinants of health: Mediating effects of caregiver mental and physical health on children's mental health. *Children and Youth Services Review, 36*, 163-169. doi: 10.1016/j.childyouth.2013.11.016.

Redinbaugh, E. M., MacCallum, R. C., & Kiecolt-Glaser, J. (1995). Recurrent syndromal depression in caregivers. *Psychology and Aging, 10*(3), 358-368. doi: 10.1037/0882-7974.10.3.358.

Rosenberg, M. (1965). *Society and the adolescent self-image*. Princeton, NJ: Princeton University Press.

Schreiner, A. S., Morimoto, T., Arai, Y., & Zarit, S. (2006). Assessing family caregiver's mental health using a statistically derived cut-off score for the Zarit burden interview. *Aging & Mental Health, 10*(2), 107-111. doi: 10.1080/13607860500312142.

Schulz, R., O'Brien, A. T., Bookwala, J., & Fleissner, K. (1995). Psychiatric and physical morbidity effects of dementia caregiving: Prevalence, correlates, and causes. *The Gerontologist, 35*(6), 771-791. doi: 10.1093/geront/35.6.771.

Schulz, R., & Sherwood, P. R. (2008). Physical and mental health effects of family caregiving. *The American Journal of Nursing, 108* (9 Suppl) (09), 23-27. doi: 10.1097/01.NAJ.0000336406.45248.4c.

Seedat, S., Scott, K. M., Angermeyer, M. C., Berglund, P., Bromet, E. J., Brugha, T. S., ... Kessler, R. C. (2009). Cross-national associations between gender and mental disorders in the World Health Organization World Mental Health Surveys. *Archives of General Psychiatry, 66*(7), 785-795. doi: 10.1001/archgenpsychiatry.2009.36.

Sperandei, S. (2014). Understanding logistic regression analysis. *Biochemia Medica, 24*(1), 12-18.

Spillman, B. C., Wolff, J., Freedman, V. A., & Kasper, J. D. (2014). *Informal caregiving for older Americans: An analysis of the 2011 National Survey of caregiving*. Washington, DC: Assistant Secretary for Planning and Evaluation.

Thompson, S. C., Bundek, N. I., & Sobolew-Shubin, A. (1990). The caregivers of stroke patients: An investigation of factors associated with depression. *Journal of Applied Social Psychology, 20*(2), 115-129. doi: 10.1111/j.1559-1816.1990.tb00402.x.

Tsai, Y., & Pai, H. (2016). Burden and cognitive appraisal of stroke survivors' informal caregivers: An assessment of depression model with mediating and moderating effects. *Archives of Psychiatric Nursing, 30*(2), 237-243. doi: 10.1016/j.apnu.2015.11.007.

United Nations, Department of Economic and Social Affairs, Population Division (2017). *World Population Ageing 2017 - Highlights* (ST/ESA/SER.A/397). Retrieved from: http://www.un.org/en/development/desa/population/publications/pdf/ageing/WPA2017_Highlights.pdf. s.f.

Vaingankar, J. A., Chong, S. A., Abdin, E., Picco, L., Jeyagurunathan, A., Zhang, Y., ... Subramaniam, M. (2016). Care participation and burden among informal caregivers of older adults with care needs and associations with dementia. *International Psychogeriatrics, 28*(2), 221-231. doi: 10.1017/S104161021500160X.

Vázquez, F. L., Otero, P., Blanco, V., López, L., & Torres, A. (2018). Psychopathological symptoms in caregivers of demented and nondemented patients. In M. Mollaoglu (Ed.), *Caregiving and Home Care* (pp. 105-124). Rikeja: Intech.

Vázquez, F. L., Torres, Á., Blanco, V., Otero, P., Díaz, O., & Ferraces, M. J. (2016). Long-term follow-up of a randomized clinical trial assessing the efficacy of a brief cognitive-behavioral depression prevention intervention for caregivers with elevated depressive symptoms. *The American Journal of Geriatric Psychiatry, 24*(6), 421-432. doi: 10.1016/j.jagp.2016.02.050.

Vos, T., Barber, R. M., Bell, B., Bertozzi-Villa, A., Biryukov, S., Bolliger, I., ... Atkins, L. S. (2015). Global, regional, and national incidence, prevalence, and years lived with disability for 301 acute and chronic diseases and injuries in 188 countries, 1990–2013: A systematic analysis for the Global Burden of Disease Study 2013. *The Lancet, 386* (9995), 743-800. doi: 10.1016/S0140-6736(15)60692-4.

Wang, M., He, B., Wang, Y., Wu, F., Chen, X., Wang, W., & Yang, X. (2016). Depression among low-income female muslim Uyghur and Kazakh informal caregivers of disabled elders in far western China: Influence on the caregivers' burden and the disabled elders' quality of life. *PLoS ONE, 11*(5), 18. doi: 10.1371/journal.pone.0156382.

Ward, R. A. (1977). The impact of subjective age and stigma on older adults". *Journal of Gerontology, 32*, 227-232.

Washington, K. T., Pike, K. C., Demiris, G., Oliver, D. P., Albright, D. L., & Lewis, A. M. (2015). Gender differences in caregiving at end of life: Implications for hospice teams. *Journal of Palliative Medicine, 18*(12), 1048-1053. doi: 10.1089/jpm.2015.0214.

Weinberger, M., Oddone, E. Z., Samsa, G. P., & Landsman, P. B. (1996). Are health-related quality-of-life measures affected by the mode of administration? *Journal of Clinical Epidemiology, 49*(2), 135–140.

Williams, A. M., Forbes, D. A., Mitchell, J., Essar, M., & Corbett, B. (2003). The influence of income on the experience of informal caregiving:

Policy implications. *Health Care for Women International, 24*(4), 280-291. doi: 10.1080/07399330303963.

Williamson, G. M., & Shaffer, D. R. (2001). Relationship quality and potentially harmful behaviors by spousal caregivers: How we were then, how we are now. *Psychology and Aging, 16*(2), 217-226. doi: 10.1037/0882-7974.16.2.217.

World Health Organization (2004). *Gender in mental health research.* Geneva: World Health Organization.

Yee, J. L., & Schulz, R. (2000). Gender differences in psychiatric morbidity among family caregivers: A review and analysis. *The Gerontologist, 40*(2), 147-164. doi: 10.1093/geront/40.2.147.

Yoon, S.-J., Kim, J.-S., Jung, J.-G., Kim, S.-S., & Kim, S. (2014). Modifiable factors associated with caregiver burden among family caregivers of terminally ill Korean cancer patients. *Supportive Care in Cancer: Official Journal of the Multinational Association of Supportive Care in Cancer*, *22*(5), 1243–1250. doi: 10.1007/s00520-013-2077-z.

Zarit, S. H., Reever, K. E., & Bach-Peterson, J. (1980). Relatives of the impaired elderly: Correlates of feelings of burden. *The Gerontologist, 20*(6), 649-655.

Zunzunegui, M., LlácerCentro, A., & Béland, F. (2002). The role of social and psychological resources in the evolution of depression in caregivers. *Canadian Journal on Aging, 21*(3), 357-369. doi: 10.1017/S0714980800001689.

In: Caregiving
Editor: Stefano Eleuteri
ISBN: 978-1-53616-889-1

Chapter 3

COSTS DERIVED FROM THE CONSUMPTION OF HEALTH RESOURCES AND LOSS OF PRODUCTIVITY IN NON-PROFESSIONAL CAREGIVERS

Fernando L. Vázquez[1], PhD, Lara López[1], MD, Vanessa Blanco[2,*], PhD, Patricia Otero[3], PhD and Ángela Torres[4], PhD

[1]Department of Clinical Psychology and Psychobiology, University of Santiago de Compostela, Santiago de Compostela, Spain
[2]Department of Evolutionary Psychology and Education, University of Santiago de Compostela, Santiago de Compostela, Spain
[3]Department of Psychology, University of A Coruña, A Coruña, Spain
[4]Department of Psychiatry, Radiology, Public Health, Nursing and Medicine, University of Santiago de Compostela, Santiago de Compostela, Spain

[*] Corresponding Author's Email: vanessa.blanco@usc.es.

ABSTRACT

Being a non-professional caregiver is associated with negative consequences at different levels. Providing care has adverse effects on physical and mental health, resulting in considerable use of health services. Caregivers also often suffer difficulties in achieving optimal performance in their paid and unpaid work. Despite these important repercussions, research on the costs related to the use of health services in this population is inconclusive. Similarly, there is hardly any data on the costs derived from impaired labor productivity as a result of health problems in caregivers. The objective of this study was to determine the most frequent health problems experienced by non-professional caregivers and to evaluate the use of health services and its predictors, direct medical costs, and indirect costs due to the loss of labor productivity. Trained psychologists collected information directly related to the study objectives from a random sample of 585 caregivers (86.8% women, mean age = 55.5 years) and administered the Trimbos/iMTA questionnaire for Costs associated with Psychiatric illness (TiC-P) to evaluate the use of medical resources and lost productivity at work. 70.6% of caregivers had used a health service in the previous three months. The services employed by the greatest proportion of caregivers were primary care physicians (59.1%), specialists (28.7%), allied health professionals (14.4%), and social workers (13.3%). The presence of chronic diseases or conditions (OR = 6.45) and symptoms of depression and anxiety (OR = 1.03) were significantly associated with an increase in the probability of using a health service. The average cost of medical services consumed, per caregiver, was €205.00 over the previous 3 months. Among caregivers with paid employment (n = 119), 16.8% were absent from work due to health problems for an average of 11.3 days in the previous month. Their reduced work efficiency resulted in a loss of 3.9 days of productivity in the previous month. This resulted in an average monthly cost of €66.47 for absences and €22.94 for reduced work efficiency per caregiver with paid employment. The majority of caregivers used health services and a significant percentage of caregivers with paid employment saw their performance affected as a result of health problems. The costs of care, in terms of medical consumption and labor productivity, must be taken into account in health care policy planning.

Keywords: caregiver, Tic-P, costs, health care resources, labor productivity

INTRODUCTION

Aging Population, Dependency, and Caregivers

The aging of the population is an unprecedented worldwide phenomenon that will continue unabated over the coming decades. Projections in the Countries of the European Union predict that people 65 years or older, who constituted 19.8% of the total population in 2018, will account for 31.3% by 2100 (Eurostat, 2019). Due to this demographic change, and to the fact that some disabling conditions are concentrated in the most elderly individuals, it is expected that the number of people who need assistance will increase. Specifically, it is expected that the number of elderly people in a situation of dependency will almost double in the Countries of the European Union, from 30.5% in 2018 to 57.3% in 2100 (Eurostat, 2019).

Given such a high percentage of people in a situation of dependency, current social and health care systems are insufficient to meet the daily needs of this population. As a consequence, most of the support these people receive comes from informal caregivers—that is, people close to the patient (usually family members, close relatives, friends, or neighbors) who provide unpaid care by performing a wide variety of tasks, including emotional support and assistance (Triantafillou et al., 2010). Informal care is already considered a fundamental component in planning long-term care and social welfare policies, given that the work carried out by caregivers is critical for maintaining social and health care systems (Rabarison et al., 2018; Reinhard, Feinberg, Choula, & Houser, 2015). However, taking care of family members is also detrimental to important aspects of caregivers' lives and, in turn, has high societal and economic costs. First, care is generally associated with a negative impact on physical and mental health (Pinquart & Sörensen, 2003; Vitaliano, Zhang, & Scanlan, 2003), which could lead to a considerable use of health resources. This is particularly true for caregivers who work, who have to juggle their own professional and family lives with their activities as carers (Eleuteri, Bellanti, & Falaschi, 2016). Second, caregivers may find it difficult to perform the tasks of both their paid and unpaid jobs (e.g., household chores, caregiving duties).

Consumption of Health Resources by Caregivers

Many caregivers suffer from multiple diseases, such as high blood pressure, back pain, joint problems, and depression and mental health issues (González-de Paz et al., 2016; Lee, Park, Matthews, & Hsieh, 2017; Perlick, Hohenstein, Clarkin, Kaczynski, & Rosenheck, 2005; Stacey, Gill, Price, & Taylor, 2018; Wang, Robinson, & Carter-Harris, 2014). Furthermore, research has also found that many conditions—including depression (Pinquart & Sörensen, 2003), arthritis (Pruchno & Potashnik, 1989), high blood pressure (Capistrant, Moon, & Glymour, 2012), back pain (Darragh et al., 2013; Suzuki, Tamakoshi, & Sakakibara, 2016), and cardiovascular events (Lee, Colditz, Berkman, & Kawachi, 2003)—are significantly more frequent in this population than in non-caregivers. A considerable body of research has examined the use of health resources in the caregiver population. However, many studies have focused on services targeted at the care recipients or support for care tasks (e.g., Hong, 2010; Toseland, McCallion, Gerber, & Banks, 2002). In studies that analyzed the frequency at which caregivers use health services (see Table 1) hospitalization rates were found to range from 4.6% in the previous 7 months (Perlick et al, 2005) to 11.7% in the previous 6 years (Zhu et al., 2015); the rate of visits to a primary care physician ranged from 10.3% in the previous 7 months (Perlick et al., 2005) to 75.8% in the previous 6 months (González-Valentín & Gálvez-Romero, 2009); outpatient visits ranged between 11.4% in the previous year (Cochrane, Goering, & Rogers, 1997) and 98.6% in the previous 3 years (Suehs et al., 2014); use of mental health professionals ranged from 8.4% in the previous month (Martindale-Adams, Nichols, Zuber, Burns, & Graney, 2016) to 30% in the previous year (Hakkaart-van Roijen et al., 2007); participation in support groups ranged from 15.7% in the previous 7 months (Perlick et al., 2015) to 16.2% in the previous month

(Martindale-Adams et al., 2016); and a rate of 12% visiting social services in the previous year (Hakkaart-van Roijen et al., 2007).

These investigations, however, provide an incomplete overview of the issue. First, the results found are heterogeneous. Although the majority of studies report the percentage of caregivers who used the particular service (e.g., Kolanowski, Fick, Waller, & Shea, 2004; Martindale-Adams et al., 2016), some only provide the average number of times that each resource was used (e.g., Bigatti & Cronan, 2002; Haley, Levine, Brown, Berry, & Hughes, 1987; Hopps, Iadeluca. McDonald, & Makinson, 2017; National Alliance for Caregiving [NAC], Schulz, & Cook, 2011; Pruchno & Potashnik, 1989), while others specify both types of results (e.g., Suehs et al., 2014; Zhu et al., 2015). Second, the majority focused on a single service or a limited number of resources (e.g., Cochrane et al., 1997; Haley et al., 1987), likely because they addressed this issue as a secondary concern and not as the main objective of the study.

In addition, when it comes to better understanding this issue, the Behavioral Model of Health Services Use (Aday & Andersen, 1974; Andersen, 1995) is one of the most widely used frameworks to detect individual factors that determine the use of health services. According to this model, there are three types of components: predisposers, which influence the propensity to use services (e.g., gender, age, educational level); enablers, which describe the individual and community means that enable the use of services (e.g., income); and need, which refers to the nature and severity of the situation of fragility (e.g., presence of diseases and chronic conditions). However, the small number of studies that have used this model in the caregiver population found mixed results. For example, Martindale-Adams et al. (2016) found that, among other variables, caregivers who were older, had a higher educational level, were married, without paid employment, with diseases, and with higher levels of depressive symptomatology used more health services for themselves. In Hong's work (2010), caregivers who used multiple care support services were more likely to be the partner of the caregiver, have fewer alternative caregivers, suffer more burden, and have more restrictions on their free time, among other factors.

Table 1. Main results of studies on the use of health services in caregivers

Study	Sample	Period	% Use (average visits)					
			Primary care physician	Outpatient	Social services	Mental health	Support groups	Hospital
Bigatti & Cronan (2002)	Fibromyalgia (*n* = 135)	1 year	(1.39)			(0.17)		(0.29)
Bremer et al. (2015)	Dementia (*N* = 1029)	1 month	31.4 %					
Cochrane et al. (1997)	Under 65 years (*N* = 1219)	1 year		11.4 %				
González-Valentín & Gálvez-Romero (2009)	In-home care (*N* = 128)	6 months	75.8 % (5.3)					5.9%
Hakkaart-van Roijen et al. (2007)	Mothers of children with ADHD (*n* = 65)	1 year	40%		12%	30%		
Haley et al. (1987)	Dementia (*n* = 44)	1 year	(2.66)					
Hopps et al. (2017)	Caregivers with paid employment (*n* = 2558)	6 months		(4.1)				(0.6)
Kolanowski et al. (2004)	Partner with dementia (*n* = 979)	3 years		75.8 %				
Martindale-Adams et al. (2016)	Dementia (*N* = 642)	1 month				8.4% (CCP)	16.2%	
Musich et al. (2017)	65 years or older (*n* = 18989)	1 year						11.3%
NAC, Schulz & Cook (2011)	Dementia (n = 583)	18 months	(114)			(33)		
Perlick et al. (2005)	Bipolar disorder (*N* = 264)	7 months	10.3 %			19.4%	15.7%	4.6%

Study	Sample	Period	% Use (average visits)					
			Primary care physician	Outpatient	Social services	Mental health	Support groups	Hospital
Pruchno & Potashnik (1989)	Dementia (*n* = 315)	1 year	(5.3)					
Schubert et al. (2008)	Alzheimer''s (*N* = 153)	6 months						10.5%
Suehs et al. (2014)	Alzheimer's (*n* = 1861)	3 years		98.6 % (61.3)				
Zhu et al. (2015)	Alzheimer's or Lewy Body Dementia (*N* = 147)	6 years		75.4 % (2.7)				11.7% (1.2)

Note. The sample sizes expressed with "N" reflect that the whole sample was analyzed; the sample sizes expressed with "n" indicate that caregivers analyzed were a subsample of the study. Not all the services analyzed are shown, due to the significant heterogeneity of resources evaluated. The values followed by the % symbol reflect the percentage of caregivers who used a particular service; values in parentheses are the average number of sessions attended. CCP = Counselor, Cleric, Psychologist.

Table 2. Costs related to the use of health services in caregivers

Study	Average cost per caregiver
Baumgarten et al. (1997)[a]	$455/1 year
Bigatti & Cronan (2002)	$1,108/1 year
Gilden et al. (2017)[a]	$694/1 month
Hakkaart-van Roijen et al. (2007)	€728/1 year
Kolanowski et al. (2004)	$4,688/3 years
Musich et al. (2017)	$945/1 month
NAC, Schulz & Cook (2011)	$6,398/1 year
Suehs et al. (2014)	$7,168/1 year
Zhu et al. (2015)	$3,068/3 years

Note. [a] = these two studies only show costs and not statistics on use

Regarding economic costs (see Table 2), the average monthly cost per caregiver ranged from $694 (Gilden, Kubisiak, Kahle-Wrobleski, Ball, & Bowman, 2017) to $945 (Musich, Wang, Kraemer, Hawkins, & Wicker,

2017), with an annual cost of between \$455 (Baumgarten et al., 1997) and \$7,168 (Suehs et al., 2014) and total three-year costs of between \$3,068 (Zhu et al., 2015) and \$4,688 (Kolanowski et al., 2004). These studies present a series of limitations. A large number focused on caregivers for people with dementia (e.g., Kolanowski et al., 2004; NAC et al., 2011; Zhu et al., 2015), and the number of resources evaluated was heterogeneous and in some cases not specified (e.g., Suehs et al., 2014). In addition, many studies employed administrative databases from large insurance companies, which may have led to errors, omissions, or problems with data quality (Suehs et al., 2014). Moreover, this estimation method makes it difficult to extrapolate the results to the Spanish context, where only 16.3% of citizens have private medical insurance (Ministry of Health, Consumer Affairs and Social Welfare, 2018).

Job Performance in Caregivers

Employment of caregivers outside of their informal caregiving may be affected to a greater or lesser extent by care tasks. This includes consequences of informal caregiving such as leaving the workforce (Covinsky et al., 2001), retiring early (de Moor et al., 2017; Longacre, Valdmanis, Handorf, & Fang, 2017), and reduction of the workdays or hours worked (Casado-Marín, García-Gómez, & López-Nicolás, 2011; de Moor et al., 2017; Schmitz & Westphal, 2017; van Houtven, Coe, & Skira, 2013). In addition, the caregiver's health status may be an additional factor that exacerbates these problems. For example, van Houtven et al. (2013) found that women caregivers in poorer health were 8% less likely to work compared to caregivers in good health. Hopps et al. (2017) found that the worsening of work performance due to health problems is significantly higher in employed caregivers than in non-caregivers. The absenteeism rate (i.e., the percentage of work time lost due to health problems in the previous week) was 8.2% in caregivers, compared to 3.6% in non-caregivers. The presenteeism rate (i.e., the percentage of time during which health problems affected productivity while working) was 24.1% in caregivers compared to 13.6% in non-caregivers. Hakkaart-van Roijen et al. (2007) found that 16%

of employed mothers of children with ADHD were absent from work due to health problems, averaging 17 days of absence per year and resulting in a cost of €1,691 per mother per year. The loss of productivity was quantified at 5 days per year, at a cost of €552. However, aside from the study by Hakkaart-van Roijen et al. (2007), we are not aware of any previous research that has analyzed the economic impact derived from this type of impairment (i.e., indirect costs) in this population.

Trimbos/iMTA Questionnaire for Costs Associated with Psychiatric Illness (TiC-P)

The use of a standardized and validated questionnaire such as the Trimbos/iMTA questionnaire for costs associated with psychiatric illnesses (Hakkaart-van Roijen, van Straten, Donker, & Tiemens, 2002) can help to rectify some of the gaps found in the literature. This instrument allows researchers to establish the direct medical costs and productivity costs derived from absences and reduced efficiency at one's paid employment. It consists of two parts: 1) assessment of medical consumption; this includes a comprehensive list of contacts with physical and mental health services; and 2) the Short Form of Health and Labor Questionnaire (SF-HLQ; van Roijen, Essink-Bot, Koopmanschap, Bonsel, & Rutten, 1996), which collects data on lost productivity in the areas of absences, reduced efficiency at work (i.e., presenteeism), and difficulties with performing one's job. This instrument has been used to assess costs associated with various problems, such as bipolar disorder (Hakkaart-van Roijen et al., 2004), minor depression (Cuijpers et al., 2007), and personality disorders (Soeteman, Hakkaart-van Roijen, Verheul, & Busschbach, 2008). Additionally, the TiC-P includes a list of 28 chronic medical diseases (e.g., migraines, cancer, rheumatic illnesses, etc.), to detect which have been experienced in the previous year. However, in relation to the caregiver population, this questionnaire has only been used in a small sample of mothers caring for children with ADHD (Hakkaart-van Roijen et al., 2007).

Purpose

The objective of this study was to analyze a sample of non-professional caregivers in terms of: (a) their use of health resources, predictors for such use, and the direct costs derived from it; (b) their absence from work, impairment of work performance and general functionality, and the indirect costs derived from these factors; and (c) which health problems they most frequently experienced.

METHODS

Participants

A cross-sectional study was conducted between January and March 2015. Participants were selected by simple random sampling from among the 18,410 informal caregivers for people in a situation of dependency collected in the official register of the regional government of Galicia (Spain). The inclusion criteria were: (a) being a family caregiver for a person whose dependence was officially recognized; (b) living with the care recipient; and (c) providing voluntary informed consent. Participants with conditions that could interfere with participation in the study (e.g., intellectual disability, significant cognitive impairment, severe visual impairment) were excluded.

The sample was estimated based on an expected indeterminate proportion (50%). Accepting an alpha risk of .05 and a 5% error rate required a total of 376 participants. Considering an expected loss rate of 40%, the sample size was increased to 627 caregivers. The response rate was 97.0%. Of the 627 caregivers invited to participate in the study, 19 (3.0%) declined the invitation. Of those that responded, 5 participants were excluded from the study and 18 did not adequately complete the evaluation. The final sample consisted of 585 caregivers (86.8% women) with an average age of 55.5 years (SD = 11.9) (see Figure 1).

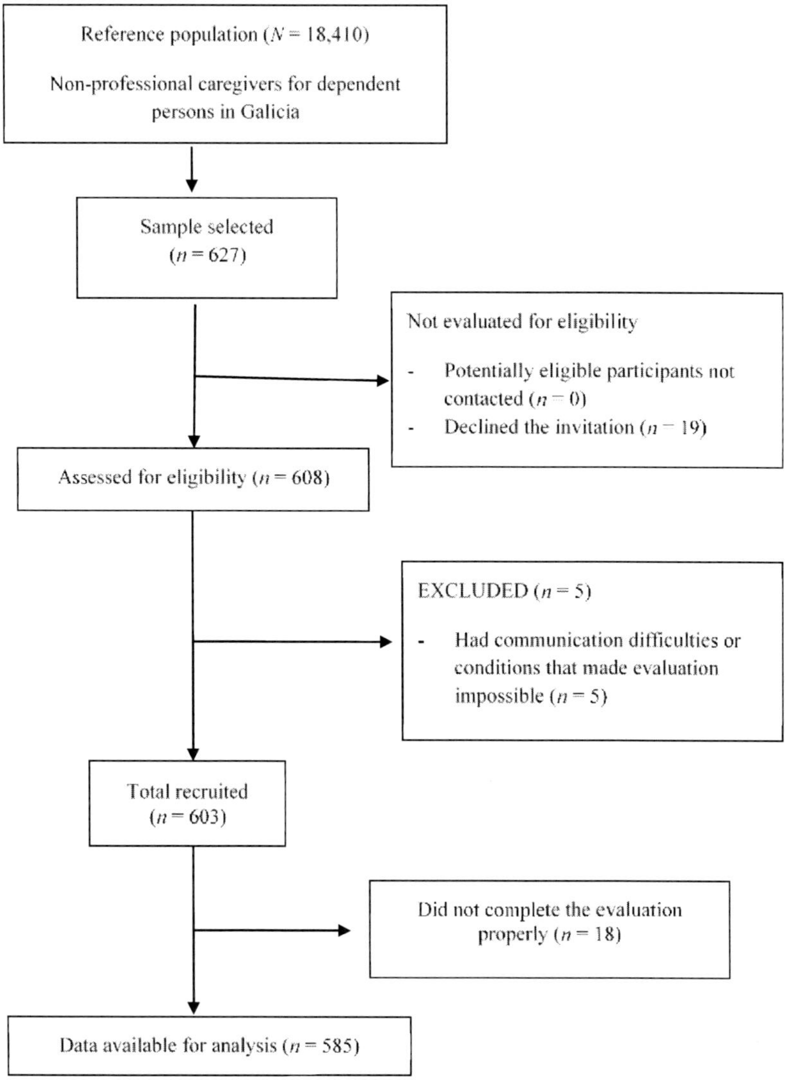

Figure 1. Flowchart of the study phases.

Participation was voluntary and no financial or other incentives were provided. All participants provided informed consent. The study respected the principles of the Declaration of Helsinki and was approved by the Bioethics Committee of the University of Santiago de Compostela.

Instruments

Caregiver Characteristics Questionnaire

The sociodemographic characteristics and the care situation were evaluated using the Caregiver Characteristics Questionnaire. This instrument was prepared ad hoc to collect information about the caregivers regarding factors potentially related to their use of health resources: (a) predisposers (i.e., sex, age, marital status, academic attainment, and relationship to the care recipient); (b) enablers (i.e., main activity, monthly income per family unit, area of residence, and support from others in providing care); and (c) need (i.e., chronic diseases and conditions, symptoms of depression and anxiety, daily hours dedicated to care, and years of providing care).

Center for Epidemiological Studies Depression Scale

Symptoms of depression and anxiety were assessed using the Center for Epidemiological Studies Depression Scale (CES-D; Radloff, 1977; Spanish version by Vázquez, Blanco, & López, 2007). The CES-D was specifically designed to detect symptoms of depression in the general population and in patients with chronic diseases (Vilagut, Forero, Barbaglia, & Alonso, 2016), but it has also been used to detect symptoms of anxiety (Dozeman et al., 2011; McQuaid, Stein, McCahill, Laffaye, & Ramel, 2000). It is a self-reported scale of 20 items with a Likert response format consisting of four options, ranging from 0 (rarely or never) to 3 (most of the time). The total score ranges from 0 to 60, with a higher score reflecting greater symptoms of depression and anxiety.

Trimbos/iMTA Questionnaire for Costs Associated with Psychiatric Illness

The use of health resources and impaired labor productivity were evaluated using the Trimbos/iMTA Questionnaire for Costs Associated with Psychiatric Illness (TiC-P; Hakkaart-van Roijen et al., 2002). This self-reported instrument consists of two parts that evaluate the consumption of health services and loss of productivity as a result of health problems. The first part of the TiC-P consists of 14 questions with a dichotomous answer format (yes/no) on the use of relevant medical resources in the previous 3 months, followed by the volume of medical consumption, and an additional question on the use of medication. It includes contacts over the previous three months with primary care services, outpatient mental health services, private and public psychiatrists, psychologists and psychotherapists, occupational health physicians, specialists, allied health professionals (physiotherapists, speech therapists), social workers, alcohol and drug rehabilitation clinics or similar institutions, alternative medicine (homeopaths, acupuncturists), self-help groups, day hospital or part-time psychiatric treatment programs, hospital admissions, medication consumption, and private medical insurance. The second part of the TiC-P includes the Short Form of Health and Labor Questionnaire (SF-HLQ; van Roijen et al., 1996), consisting of three modules that measure lost productivity during the previous month due to health problems: absence from work, reduced efficiency, and difficulties in work performance. Absence from work is evaluated in terms of the number of days of absence due to health problems in the previous month and months of leave (if the respondent has been absent for more than one month). For reduced efficiency, respondents indicate the number of days that were worked during the previous month despite having health problems and give them a performance score that ranges from 1 (performance much worse than normal) to 10 (normal performance). The instrument then presents 7 items that assess the frequency of the problems constituting this reduced efficiency: concentration, pace of work, need to work in isolation, decision-making, postponement of work, delegation of work, and others (an open-ended question). The response options range from 1 (never) to 4 (almost always). Then the instrument asks the amount of overtime needed to compensate for work lost due to health problems and the respondent's monthly net salary from their job. Finally, it assesses the degree of difficulty in performing four categories of unpaid work (household chores, shopping, minor home repairs, and activities with children), with response options ranging from 0 (no hindrance) to 2 (significant hindrance). Additionally, it includes a list of 28 chronic diseases and conditions, with the respondent indicating which they have experienced in the previous year. It takes approximately 10 minutes to complete the questionnaire and the instrument has an acceptable test-retest reliability and construct validity for the evaluated items (Bouwmans et al., 2013).

Procedure

To standardize the evaluation, a research protocol was developed that details the objectives of the study, its design and framework, the participants (sampling, eligibility criteria, and recruitment), its measures, biases (non-response, recall, selection), quality control for the procedure, data management and analysis, and ethical aspects.

Before the study, a pilot study was conducted with 30 randomly selected caregivers to assess the adequacy of the assessment instruments, the competence of the evaluators, and the feasibility of the project. Subsequently, the selected caregivers were contacted via letter informing them of the study and asking them to return a sealed postcard if they did not wish to participate. Those who did not return the card were contacted by phone and those who were interested were invited to participate. To minimize the loss of participants, the researchers followed the recommended strategies for this type of study, such as providing written information in advance, reminders of the interview date, eliminating invasive data collection procedures, and presenting the study in an appealing manner (Hulley, Cummings, Browner, Grady, & Newman, 2013). The previously trained evaluators presented the self-administered evaluation instruments at sites close to the participants' homes. Each evaluation took approximately 30 minutes.

Data Analysis

The statistical package SPSS for Windows (version 24.0) and Excel 2016 (Microsoft, Redmond, WA, USA) were used to analyze the data.

Frequencies, percentages, means, and standard deviations were calculated for the caregiver variables of *predisposers*, *enablers*, and *need*.

Use of Health Services and Predictors

Descriptive and frequency statistics were applied to assess the use of health services. The exception was item 2, which assesses consultation visits to regional outpatient mental health service providers (RIAGG), which do not exist in Spain. This function is handled by public and private psychiatrists and psychologists.

A multivariate logistic regression analysis was then performed to evaluate associations between the use of a service (dependent variable: 0 = no, 1 = yes) and caregivers' predisposing, enabling and need variables (potential predictors). The variables with a $p \leq .30$ in the bivariate analyses were incorporated into the multivariate logistic regression analysis to determine the adjusted relationship between the predictive variables and the use of services. The results were reported as adjusted odds ratios (OR) with 95% confidence intervals (CI).

Direct Costs

Direct costs were defined as the monetary value of the resources used to diagnose and treat medical problems. Decree 56/2014 was used to determine the unit cost of each service. This decree establishes the rates for health services provided in centers that are part of the Galician Health Care Service and in public health foundations that set prices per visit and the cost per bed and per night for in-patient services. The unit costs per visit with private psychiatrists/psychologists, physicians at work, alternative medicine providers, self-help groups, and private medical insurance are not subject to specific regulations and so the authors themselves estimated these costs through a query of notable professionals in these areas. The estimate of Salvador-Carulla et al. (2011) was used to set the unit cost per visit with a social worker. In calculating costs, visits were considered as check-ups/follow-ups (not initial consultations), with the understanding that given the average age of the caregivers, they would be patients with an ongoing

Table 3. Predisposing, enabling and need characteristics of the sample (N = 585)

Characteristics	*n* (%)
Predisposers	
Caregiver sex	
Male	77 (13.2)
Female	508 (86.8)
Age	
M	55.5
SD	11.9
Partner	
Without partner	163 (27.9)
With partner	422 (72.1)
Level of education	
No schooling	88 (15.0)
Primary	314 (53.7)
Secondary/University	183 (31.3)
Relationship	
Other	519 (88.7)
Partner	66 (11.3)
Enablers	
Occupation	
No paid employment	466 (79.7)
Paid employment	119 (20.3)
Monthly income	
Up to €999	145 (24.8)
From €1000 to €1999	337 (57.6)
€2000 or more	103 (17.6)
Area of residence	
Rural	228 (39.0)
Urban	357 (61.0)
Help with care	
No	276 (47.2)
Yes	309 (52.8)
Need	
Daily hours of care	
M	15.7
SD	4.2
Years caring	
M	13.3
SD	9.5
Depressive and anxiety symptomatology	
M	18.0
SD	11.3
Chronic diseases	
No	157 (26.8)
Yes	428 (73.2)

history in the health care system. Likewise, given the difference in costs between psychiatric and psychology professionals and the absence of disaggregated data, the average cost of unit costs for a visit with a psychiatrist or psychologist was calculated for the items related to visits to private psychiatrists and psychologists (item 3) and public providers of the same type (item 4). The average cost per caregiver was determined by multiplying the average number of visits attended per caregiver (not per service user) by the unit cost. The percentage of cost per caregiver in the previous 3 months was calculated by dividing the average cost of that service by the average total cost per caregiver. Total costs were calculated by summing the average cost per caregiver for each of the services.

The item on medication use, doses, and frequencies included a great deal of data and many incorrect and incomplete responses. Given that only 2.4% of caregivers were taking medications, we decided to follow the same course of action used by Timman, Bouwmans, Busschbach, and Hakkaart-van Roijen (2015) in dealing with a similar problem—that is, to exclude medication costs from the analysis.

Indirect Costs

Indirect costs due to work absences were obtained by multiplying the average days of absence during the last 3 months by the net cost per day (average monthly net salary x 12/365). To collect data on the reduction in work efficiency, participants with paid employment were asked to estimate the amount of overtime they would have had to work to offset the health-related loss of productivity they had experienced in the previous month. Costs derived from days of absence from work and hours lost at work due to health-related problems were assessed using net income per day.

Results

Sociodemographic and Clinical Characteristics

Table 3 shows the characteristics of the sample, classified according to the Behavioral Model on the Use of Health Services. The final sample was composed of 585 caregivers, who were predominantly women (86.8%), with an average age of 55.5 years (*SD* = 11.9). The majority had a partner (72.1%), had completed primary education (53.7%), and provided care for relatives other than their partner (88.7%). In addition, the majority did not have paid employment (79.7%), had a monthly family income that ranged between €1,000 and €1,999 (57.6%), lived in an urban area (61.0%), and had other people to help them with their care tasks (52.8%). The average daily time spent providing care was 15.7 hours (*SD* = 4.2), and they had been providing care for an average of 13.3 years (*SD* = 9.5). The average score on the CES-D scale was 18.0 (*SD* = 11.3), and the majority had at least one illness (73.2%).

Use of Health Services and Predictors

As Table 4 shows, 70.6% of caregivers reported having used some type of health resource in the previous three months. Specifically, 59.1% had visited their primary care physician. Among those who made visits, the average was 3.0 visits (*SD* = 2.6) during the previous three months. Among the participants, 28.7% had visited a specialist, with an average consumption of 2.5 sessions (*SD* = 2.5). Meanwhile, 14.4% had visited an allied health professional, making an average of 6.5 visits (*SD* = 6.6) during the last three months. Social worker services had been used by 13.3%, attending an average of 2.0 meetings (*SD* = 1.8). The rest of the services evaluated were used by less than 7% of caregivers: alternative medicine services (6.5%), public (5.0%) and private psychiatrists/ psychologists (4.8%), self-help groups (4.4%), occupational physicians (2.4%), and hospitalizations (1.2%). A small percentage (2.4%) reported that they were taking medication, and 0.5% had private medical insurance. None of the caregivers had visited an alcohol or drug rehabilitation clinic or participated in a day hospitalization or part-time psychiatric treatment program.

Table 5 shows the results of the multivariate logistic regression analysis in relation to the factors associated with the use of services. The final model explained 26.6% of the data and presented an adequate goodness of fit (x^2

Hosmer and Lemeshow (8) = 11.48; $p = .18$). It correctly classified 77.1% of the cases, with high sensitivity (86.7%) but low specificity (54.1%). None of the predisposing and enabling variables included were significantly associated with the use of services. With respect to the need variables, the presence of chronic diseases or conditions (OR = 6.45, 95% CI 4.21-9.87) and symptoms of depression and anxiety (OR = 1.03, 95% CI 1.01-1.05) were significantly associated with an increase in the probability of using a health resource.

Table 4. Use and costs of health resources in the previous three months (*N* = 585)

Service	Utilization	Assistance per user	Cost per unit (€)	Average cost per caregiver (€)	% cost over the last 3 months
	N (%)	*M (SD)*			
Primary care	346 (59.1)	3.0 (2.6)	34.62[1]	61.28	29.9
Public psychiatrist, psychologist	29 (5.0)	2.6 (2.7)	41.63[1]	5.41	2.6
Private psychiatrist, psychologist	28 (4.8)	2.8 (3.4)	80.00[2]	10.72	5.2
Doctor at workplace	14 (2.4)	3.3 (1.5)	70.00[2]	5.60	2.7
Specialist	168 (28.7)	2.5 (2.5)	58.37[1]	42.03	20.5
Allied health professional	84 (14.4)	6.5 (6.6)	21.14[1]	19.66	9.6
Social worker	78 (13.3)	2.0 (1.8)	49.10[3]	13.26	6.5
Alcohol and drug clinic	0 (0.0)				
Alternative medicine	38 (6.5)	4.4 (5.3)	50.00[2]	14.50	7.1
Self-help	26 (4.4)	3.8 (4.6)	0.00[2]	0	
Day hospital or part-time psychiatric treatment program	0 (0.0)			0	
Hospitalization	7 (1.2)	5.1 (4.8)	528.95[1]	31.74	15.5
Medication consumption	14 (2.4)				
Private medical insurance	3 (0.5)	1 (assumed)	80.70[2]	0.807	0.4
They used some service	413 (70.6)				
Total				205.00	

Note. Source: [1]Decree 56/2014, which establishes rates for health services provided in centers that are part of the Galician Health Service and public health care foundations, 2014, April 30. [2] Authors' estimate based on the average of the rates for private services in our context. [3] Salvador-Carulla et al. (2011)

Table 5. Results of logistic regression analyses on the use of services

	B	SE	Wald	*p*	OR	95% CI	
						Lower	Upper
Predisposers							
Caregiver sex							
Male	1 [Reference]						
Female	0.17	0.30	0.32	.571	1.19	0.66	2.14
Caregiver age	0.01	0.01	1.00	.316	1.01	0.99	1.03
Enablers							
Monthly income							
Up to €999	1 [Reference]						
From €1000 to €1999	0.33	0.24	1.87	.172	1.39	0.87	2.25
€2000 or more	0.45	0.33	1.87	.172	1.56	0.82	2.97
Help with care							
No	1 [Reference]						
Yes	- 0.33	0.21	2.42	.120	0.72	0.47	1.09
Need							
Chronic diseases							
No	1 [Reference]						
Yes	1.86	0.22	73.63	< .001	6.45	4.21	9.87
Depressive and anxiety symptomatology	0.03	0.01	6.72	0.10	1.03	1.01	1.05
Daily hours of care	0.01	0.03	0.10	.755	1.01	0.96	1.06
Years caring	0.01	0.01	0.51	.474	1.01	0.99	1.03
R^2 Nagelkerke	.266						
X^2 Hosmer and Lemeshow	11.48 (8); $p = .176$						

Note. B = regression coefficient; SE: Standard error; Wald = Wald statistic; *p* = level of significance; OR = Odds Ratio; 95% CI = 95% Confidence Interval of 95%

Direct and Indirect Costs

Table 4 shows the direct costs for the previous 3 months, for each service. Direct medical costs per caregiver during the last 3 months were €205.00. The cost of primary care accounted for 29.9% of the cost, followed by the costs of specialists (20.5%) and hospitalization (15.5%). The rest of the services, considered individually, accounted for less than 10% of the total cost: allied health professionals (9.6%), alternative medicine (7.1%), social workers (6.5%), private psychiatrists and psychologists (5.2%), occupational physicians (2.7%), public psychiatrists and psychologists (2.6%), and the cost of medical insurance (0.4%).

Regarding indirect costs, 20.3% of caregivers (*n* = 119) had paid employment, earning an average net salary of €1,065.30 per month for a workday that averaged 6.3 hours per day. For those with paid employment, 16.8% (*n* = 20) were absent from work due to health problems in the previous month, for an average of 11.3 days (*SD* = 12.3). The periods of absence were relatively long, because 45% (*n* = 9) were on leave for more than one month due to health problems, with an average of 5.7 months (*SD* = 5.3). The average monthly cost due to absences from work was €66.47 per working caregiver. Those who experienced reduced efficiency at work (*n* = 20) experienced an average loss of productivity during the previous month of approximately 24.4 hours (*SD* = 33.8), which would be equivalent to 3.9 workdays (considering half of a 6.3-hour workday). The associated average monthly cost was €22.94 per caregiver with paid employment (see Table 6).

Caregivers with paid employment whose performance was affected by health problems in the previous month (*n* = 20), gave their performance an average score of 6.6 out of 10 (*SD* = 1.5). As a result of health problems, 55.0% said they "sometimes" had concentration problems, 65.0% said they "sometimes" had to work more slowly, and 55.0% said they "sometimes" had occasions when they went to their job but had more difficulty making decisions. Moreover, 75.0% "almost never" had to work in isolation, 55.0% "almost never" had to postpone work, 75.0% "almost never" had to have other people take over their work, and 100.0% indicated they "almost never" had other problems. The average efficiency score was 10.6 (*SD* = 3.5).

Table 6. Average number of days lost due to absence from work, reduced efficiency, and indirect costs of caregivers (*n* = 119)

Type of loss of productivity	Duration	Costs (in euros)	Total cost per caregiver with paid employment
Absence from work (*n* = 20)	11.3 days	Net per day: 35.0	66.47
Reduced efficiency (*n* = 20)	3.9 days		22.94
Total	15.2		89.41

Table 7. Chronic conditions and diseases in the previous year (*N* = 585)

Condition	*n*	%[a]
Chronic back problems (more than 3 months) or herniated disc	197	33.7
Joint inflammation (osteoarthritis) of the hands or feet.	121	20.7
High blood pressure	107	18.3
Joint deterioration (arthritis) of the knees, hips, or hands.	86	14.7
Overexertion, depression, severe nervousness.	86	14.7
Migraine	77	13.2
Thyroid disease	55	9.4
Dizziness and falls	46	7.9
Other rheumatic diseases lasting more than 3 months.	45	7.7
Asthma, chronic bronchitis or Chronic Obstructive Pulmonary Disease.	43	7.4
Diabetes	36	6.2
Infection of the nasal cavity, frontal sinus or others.	34	5.8
Chronic skin disease or eczema.	32	5.5
Injury due to an accident at home, while playing sports, at work or traffic accident.	30	5.1
Gastric or duodenal ulcer	20	3.4
Severe heart disease or heart attack.	19	3.2
Severe intestinal disorders of more than 3 months duration	19	3.2
Kidney stones	19	3.2
Gallstones or gallbladder infection	16	2.7
Cancer	13	2.2
Prolapse	7	1.2
Severe kidney disease	6	1.0
Liver infection or cirrhosis of the liver	5	0.9
Chronic bladder infection	5	0.9
Stroke, or the consequences of a stroke	3	0.5
Epilepsy.	3	0.5
Other neurological diseases, such as Parkinson's disease.	3	0.5
Multiple sclerosis.	1	0.2

Note. [a] % = the sum of the categories exceeds 100% because they are not mutually exclusive

For all caregivers (*n* = 585), in relation to difficulties in performing unpaid work, the percentage of caregivers who experienced "some kind of problem" was 43.9% for performing household chores, 41.2% for going shopping, 57.4% for doing odd jobs at home, and 20.6% for taking care of children.

Health Problems

As Table 7 shows, caregivers in the sample most frequently reported symptoms of chronic back problems or herniated disc (33.7%), followed by osteoarthritis of the hands or feet (20.7%), high blood pressure (18.3%), arthritis in the knees, hips, or hands (14.7%) and overexertion, depression, and serious nervousness (14.7%).

Discussion

Main Findings

The objective of this study was to evaluate non-professional caregivers' use of health services and their predictors, direct medical costs, and indirect costs due to a loss of productivity at work. In the previous three months, caregivers most frequently used the services of primary care physicians, specialists, allied health professionals, and social workers. The average cost of medical consumption per caregiver was €205. Out of the caregivers with paid employment (around 1 in 5 of the total), 20% had to be absent from work due to health problems for about one-third of the month, and their loss of productivity was about 4 days in the previous month. This resulted in an average cost of approximately €66 for absenteeism and €23 for loss of productivity, for a total cost of approximately €89 per month. The most frequently self-reported medical problems were chronic back problems, osteoarthritis of the hands or feet, and high blood pressure.

The Broader Context

In our study, the percentage of caregivers who visited a primary care physician in the previous 3 months (59.1%) was slightly lower than that found in a study among Spanish caregivers (González-Valentín & Gálvez-

Romero, 2009) that reported that 75.8% of the sample visited a primary care physician in the previous 6 months. However, it was higher than the 40% of caregivers visiting a primary care physician by Hakkaart-van Roijen et al. (2007), the 31.4% by Bremer et al. (2015), or the 10.3% in the previous 7 months that Perlick et al. (2005) found. The differences found in the findings of studies conducted in other countries may be due to the configuration of the Spanish health system, where primary care plays a very prominent role.

Visits to specialists, which 28.7% of caregivers reporting having made in the previous three months, were less frequent than that found in the studies by Kolanowski et al. (2004), Suehs et al. (2014) and Zhu et al. (2015). However, these studies evaluated this resource together with others (such as primary care) and did not provide disaggregated data, which explains the considerably higher numbers of outpatient visits. Nevertheless, the percentage found in the present study is higher than that reported by Cochrane et al. (1997), who found that 11.4% of caregivers had visited a specialist in the previous year. Compared to previous research that used the TiC-P in samples that included mental health conditions (e.g., Hakkaart-van Roijen et al., 2004; Soeteman et al., 2008), the percentage found in our investigation is higher (28.7% in three months vs. 10% and 10.1% per year, respectively).

On the other hand, the frequency of caregivers who visited allied health professionals (14.4%) is similar to figures found in previous research: 10% (Hakkaart-van Roijen et al., 2004) and 11.9% in the previous year (Soeteman et al., 2008). The use of social services in our work (13.3%) was also very similar to the figure found by Hakkaart-van Roijen et al. (2007) in the previous year (12%).

The use of mental health resources (9.8%, considering public and private professionals) is lower than findings in other works, such as Perlick et al. (2005), who found that 19.4% of caregivers had received individual outpatient psychotherapy in the previous 7 months. However, this difference may be due to the fact that the caregivers in the Perlick et al. (2005) sample were recruited when their family members were admitted to a hospital with a diagnosis of bipolar disorder, and thus medical professionals may have been more attentive to the caregivers' emotional state and have referred them more frequently to this service.

The frequency of use of support groups (4.4%) was lower than the findings of Perlick et al. (2005; 15.7% in the previous 7 months) and Martindale-Adams et al. (2016; 16% in the previous month). This latter study used baseline data from a randomized controlled trial, and so the sample may have been composed of participants with high stress levels and burden who were more likely to participate in an intervention study. Another possible explanation is that finding emotional support through self-help groups is an approach not widely used in our context.

The frequency at which caregivers had been hospitalized in the previous 3 months (1.2%) was lower in our study than in most studies that also explored this issue, such as the 5.9% in the previous 6 months that González-Valentín & Gálvez-Romero (2009) reported, 4.6% in the previous 7 months reported by Perlick et al. (2005), 11.3% over the previous year reported by Musich et al. (2017); 10.5% over the previous 6 months reported by Schubert et al. (2008); and 11.7% in the previous 6 months reported by Zhu et al. (2015).

The use of alternative medicine (6.3%) was lower than that found in populations with mental health conditions that also completed TiC-P, such as Hakkaart-van Roijen et al. (2004), who reported a utilization rate of 12.5% per year, and Soeteman et al. (2008), where that same statistic was 10.9% per year.

Regarding visits to an occupational physician, our findings (2.4%) were similar to the 2.5% per year rate in people with bipolar disorder (Hakkaart-van Roijen et al., 2004), but lower than the 9% per year in mothers of children with ADHD (Hakkaart-van Roijen et al., 2007), and 25.1% per year in people with personality disorders (Soeteman et al., 2008).

Analyzing the factors associated with the use of services based on the Behavioral Model on the Use of Health Services showed that, with respect to the need variables, the presence of diseases or chronic conditions (OR = 6.45) and symptoms of depression and anxiety (OR = 1.03) were significantly associated with an increase in the probability of using health resources. This is consistent with Martindale-Adams et al. (2016) and Hong

(2010). The latter study found a greater likelihood of the use of services in those caregivers who reported a greater burden. Thus, although they evaluate different predisposing, enabling and need variables, these studies tend to coincide in finding a greater use of resources by caregivers who suffer from diseases or high levels of emotional distress. These findings add support to the need to provide effective measures that reduce caregivers' physical and mental burdens and thus reduce the consumption of health resources.

As previously noted, our study found that direct medical costs averaged €205 per caregiver over the previous 3 months. These figures are similar to those of some studies of caregivers (e.g., Baumgarten et al., 1997; Bigatti & Cronan, 2002; Hakkaart-van Roijen et al., 2007; Kolanowski et al., 2004; Zhu et al., 2015), but they are lower compared to other investigations (Gilden et al., 2017; Musich et al., 2017; NAC et al., 2011, Suehs et al., 2014). Overall, studies that used the TiC-P in non-caregiver samples found results in a similar range (e.g., €434/year in Acarturk et al., 2009; €728/year in Hakkaart-van Roijen et al., 2004). However, the study by Soeteman et al. (2008) found a higher cost (€7,398 per year), probably because it focused on participants with personality disorders who were receiving professional help at the time of the study. Various factors may explain the discrepancies compared to the rest of the studies. On one hand, we must look at the resources included in determining costs: some studies included medication expenses (NAC et al., 2011), while others included expenses for specific services, such as transportation, medical equipment, and testing (e.g., Gilden et al., 2017). On the other hand, there is also a wide range of variation in the prices for services between different countries. In fact, this phenomenon is the source of geographic variation most frequently cited in economic studies of health care (Sculpher et al., 2004). Thus, for example, most of the studies that used the TiC-P focused on Dutch samples, whose guidelines set higher unit prices than those used in this chapter (see the latest price update in Tan, Bouwmans, Rutten, & Hakkaart-van Roijen, 2012).

With respect to indirect costs, our study found that among caregivers with paid employment (n = 119), approximately 17% suffered job performance problems. Specifically, in the previous month they reported an average of approximately 11 days of absence and a reduction in efficiency of around 4 days. These figures are similar to those found in mothers taking care of children with ADHD for a period of one full year (Hakkaart-van Roijen et al., 2007), with respect to days of absence (17 days) and reduced efficiency (5 days), but are lower than those found in people with bipolar disorder for a time frame of one year, during which days of absence averaged 55.5 and reduced efficiency was 7.7 days (Hakkaart-van Roijen et al., 2004). They are also lower than the figures reported in a study population of persons with personality disorders, who reported an average of 47.6 days of absence per year (Soeteman et al., 2008). On the other hand, the associated costs calculated in our study (€66.47 and €22.94/month) are much lower than the cost of €2,243 per year found in the study of mothers taking care of children with ADHD (Hakkart-van Roijen et al., 2007), US$3,109 per year in people with minor depression (Cuijpers et al., 2007), €7,088 per year in people with personality disorders (Soeteman et al., 2008), and €5,331 per year in people with social anxiety (Acarturk et al., 2009). These apparently contradictory results may be due to the disparity in the methods used to establish the value of hours worked and the inclusion of hours of household labor in the calculations (e.g., Cuijpers et al., 2007). Regarding the difficulties of conducting their work, the most frequently affected work areas were concentration (55%), pace of work (65%), and decision-making (65%). This contrasts with the study by Hakkaart-van Roijen et al. (2007), where the most frequent difficulty was having to work in isolation (36%). Both studies agree that a minority had to postpone work. Efficiency scores were also similar (10.6 vs. 13.0 in Hakkaart-van Roijen et al., 2007).

Difficulties in performing unpaid tasks were more intense in our sample: approximately 21% to 57% had some type of problem in performing childcare tasks, minor home repairs, going shopping, or doing housework. Hakkaart-van Roijen et al. (2007) reported that 20% of the mothers had experienced problems in the performance of unpaid tasks and only specified that 12% had difficulties in childcare.

The most frequent medical conditions that caregivers experienced during the previous year were back problems, osteoarthritis, high blood pressure, arthritis, overexertion, depression, and severe nervousness. These findings are consistent with those reported in other studies, where these types of diseases are at the top of the lists of medical conditions most frequently self-reported by caregivers (e.g., Lee et al., 2017; Wang et al., 2014; Perlick et al., 2005; Stacey et al., 2018; González-de Paz et al., 2016). In addition, many of these conditions, such as back pain (Suzuki et al., 2016), high blood pressure (Capistrant et al., 2012), and mental health problems (Pinquart & Sorensen, 2003) have been found to be significantly related to the care situation.

Strengths and Limitations

This chapter presents a series of strengths. First, it adds evidence about the economic implications of two areas frequently related to health status in non-professional caregivers: medical consumption and work performance. In addition, it uses a standardized and validated instrument that allows researchers to obtain results that are comparable between studies and that offers a comprehensive evaluation of these issues, thereby reducing the probability of yielding incomplete evaluations. Moreover, the response rate was very high (97.0%), producing a large and representative sample (N = 585). However, this study also has some limitations. First, its cross-sectional nature prevents inference of a causal relationship between the care situation and the results. Future studies should include a comparison group to analyze excess costs and should adopt a longitudinal perspective (i.e., periodic follow-ups) to analyze the pattern of service use and work trajectories as the care recipient's disease progresses. Second, the cost calculations were based on self-reported indicators, and thus the responses may have suffered from recall bias. However, a recent meta-analysis (Leggett et al., 2016) found that self-report questionnaires (including the TiC-P) constitute a valid method for collecting data on the use of health services. Finally, the different time periods used in the existing literature to measure the costs of health services and loss of productivity at work have hindered comparability among results. To overcome this limitation, previous work (Hakkaart-van Roijen et al., 2007) has inferred the use of services on an annualized basis according to the frequency of service utilization over different measurement time periods.

The cost-friction method has also been used to estimate productivity costs derived from health problems, calculating the value of lost productivity during the period of friction (i.e., between the beginning of the loss of labor time or productivity and the time of labor replacement). The absence of several evaluation points (due to the cross-sectional design) and the absence of Spanish data on the period of friction prevented an estimation of the results on an annualized basis, which would perhaps improve the comparability of our findings.

Implications for Clinical, Political, and Research Practice

The results of this chapter have important implications for clinical practice and health policies aimed at the provision of care for people in situations of dependency. The labor that caregivers assume is crucial, both for care recipients and for the maintenance of societal and health care systems because their replacement with formal care services is not economically feasible or socially desirable (Hoffmann & Rodrigues, 2010). In addition, sociodemographic trends indicate that their labor will be even more important in the future, but also more complicated: the progressive incorporation of women into the labor market and the reduction in the size of nuclear families will increase the burden experienced by these caregivers. Therefore, measures must be planned to ensure that caregivers achieve a balance between the tasks of caring, their well-being, and their working lives. This implies understanding the consequences they suffer due to their efforts. Along these lines, this study adds evidence on the patterns of use of a wide range of health resources, as well as the deterioration in working caregivers' jobs and general productivity. The results on the individual determinants for the use of health services underscore the importance of paying special attention to those caregivers who have medical conditions or high levels of depression/anxiety symptoms. In addition, the economic implications shown in this paper suggest that the costs of care should be included in political discussions and health policy planning.

Conclusion

This study shows that most caregivers are utilizers of health services and a significant percentage of caregivers with paid employment suffer from reduced work performance as a result of their health problems. The costs of care in terms of consumption of health resources and impairment of labor productivity should be included when planning care policies over the long term.

References

Acarturk, C., Smit, F., de Graaf, R., van Straten, A., ten Have, M. & Cuijpers, P. (2009). Economic costs of social phobia: a population-based study. *Journal of Affective Disorders*, *115*, 421-429. doi:10.1016/ j.jad.2008.10.008.

Aday, L. A. & Andersen, R. (1974). A framework for the study of access to medical care. *Health Services Research*, *9*, 208-220.

Andersen, R. M. (1995). Revisiting the Behavioral Model and Access to Medical Care; Does it Matter? *Journal of Health and Social Behavior*, *36*, 1-10.

Baumgarten, M., Battista, R. N., Infante-Rivard, C., Hanley, J. A., Becker, R., Bilker, W. B. & Gauthier, S. (1997). Use of physician services among family caregivers of elderly persons with Dementia. *Journal of Clinical Epidemiology*, *11*, 1265-1272.

Bigatti, S. M. & Cronan, T. A. (2002). An examination of the physical health, health care use, and psychological well-being of spouses of people with fibromyalgia syndrome. *Health Psychology*, *21*, 157-166. doi:10.1037//0278-6133.21.2.157.

Bouwmans, C., de Jong, K., Timman, R., Zijlstra-Vlasveld, M., van der Feltz-Cornelis, C., Tan Swan, S. & Hakkaart-van Roijen, L. (2013). Feasibility, reliability and validity of a questionnaire on healthcare consumption and productivity loss in patients with a psychiatric disorder

(TiC-P). *BMC Health Services Research*, *13*, 217. doi:10.1186/1472-6963-13-217.

Bremer, P., Cabrera, E., Leino-Kilpi, H., Lethin, C., Saks, K., Sutcliffe, C. & Wübker, A. (2015). Informal dementia care: consequences for caregivers' health and health care use in 8 European countries. *Health Policy*, *119*, 1459-1471. doi: 10.1016/j.healthpol.2015.09.014.

Capistrant, B. D., Moon J. R. & Glymour, M. M. (2012). Spousal caregiving and incident hypertension. *American Journal of Hypertension*, *25*, 1-14. doi:10.1038/ajh.2011.232.

Casado-Marín, D., García-Gómez, P. & López-Nicolás, Á. (2011). Informal care and labour force participation among middle-aged women in Spain. *SERIEs*, *2*, 1-29.

Cochrane, J. J., Goering, P. N. & Rogers, J. (1997). The mental health of informal caregivers in Ontario: an epidemiological survey. *American Journal of Public Health*, *87*, 2002-2007.

Covinsky, K. E., Eng, K., Lui, L., Sand, L. P., Sehgal, A. R., Walter, L. C. & Yaffe, K. (2001). Reduced Employment in Caregivers of Frail Elders: Impact of Ethnicity, Patient Clinical Characteristics, and Caregiver Characteristics. *Journal of Gerontology: Medical Sciences*, *56A*, M707-M713.

Cuijpers, P., Smit, F., Oostenbrink, J., de Graaf, R., ten Have, M. & Beekman, A. (2007). Economic costs of minor depression: a population-based study. *Acta Psychiatrica Scandinavica*, *115*, 229-236. doi:10.1111/j.1600-0447.2006.00851.x.

Darragh, A. R., Sommerich, C. M., Lavender, S. A., Tanner, K. J., Voger, K. & Campo, M. (2013). Musculoskeletal Discomfort, Physical Demand, and Caregiving Activities in Informal Caregivers. *Journal of Applied Gerontology*, *34*, 734-760. doi:10.1177/0733464813496464.

de Moor, J. S., Dowling, E. C., Ekwueme, D. U., Guy, G. P., Rodriguez, J., Virgo, K. S. & Yabroff, K. R. (2017). Employment implications of informal cancer caregiving. *Journal of Cancer Survivorship*, *11*, 48-57. doi:10.1007/s11764-016-0560-5.

Decreto 56/2014, por el que se establecen las tarifas de los servicios sanitarios prestados en los centros dependientes del Servicio Gallego de

Salud y en las fundaciones públicas sanitarias [Decree 56/2014, which establishes the rates of the health services provided in the centers dependent on the Galician Health Service and in the public health foundations]. (2014, 30 de abril). Diario Oficial de Galicia [DOG], 96, 21 de mayo, 2014. Retrieved from: https://www.xunta.gal/dog/Publicados/2014/20140521/AnuncioC3K1-140514-0001_es.pdf.

Dozeman, E., van Schaik, D. J., van Marwijk, H. W., Stek, M. L., van der Horst, H. E. & Beekman, A. T. (2011). The center for epidemiological studies depression scale (CES-D) is an adequate screening instrument for depressive and anxiety disorders in a very old population living in residential homes. *International Journal of Geriatric Psychiatry*, *26*, 239–246. doi: 10.1002/gps.2519.

Eleuteri, S., Bellanti, G. & Falaschi, P. (2016). Hip fracture: preliminary results supporting significant correlations between the psychological wellbeing of patients and their relative caregivers. *Journal of Gerontology & Geriatrics*, *64*, 104-111.

Eurostat (2019*). Population structure and ageing*. Retrieved from: https://ec.europa.eu/eurostat/statistics-explained/index.php/ Population_structure_and_ageing.

Gilden, D. M., Kubisiak, J. M., Kahle-Wrobleski, K., Ball, D. E. & Bowman, L. (2017). A Claims-Based Examination of Health Care Costs Among Spouses of Patients with Alzheimer's Disease. *Journals of Gerontology: Medical Sciences*, *72*, 811-817. doi:10.1093/gerona/ glx029.

González-de Paz, L., Real, J., Borrás-Santos, A., Martínez-Sánchez, J. M., Rodrigo-Baños, V. & Navarro-Rubio, M. D. (2016). Associations between informal care, disease, and risk factors: A Spanish country-wide population-based study. *Journal of Public Health Policy*, *37*, 173-189. doi:10.1057/jphp.2016.3.

González-Valentín, A. & Gálvez-Romero, C. (2009). Características sociodemográficas, de salud y utilización de recursos sanitarios de cuidadores de ancianos atendidos en domicilio [Socio-demographic characteristics of health and use of sanitary resources by elderly caregivers at home]. *Gerokomos*, *20*, 15-21

Hakkaart-van Roijen, L., Hoeijenbos, M. B., ten Have, M., Nolen, W. A., Veraart, C. P. W. M. & Rutten, F. F. H. (2004). The societal costs and quality of life of patients suffering from bipolar disorder in the Netherlands. *Acta Psychiatrica Scandinavica*, *110*, 383–392.

Hakkaart-van Roijen, L., van Straten, A., Donker, M. & Tiemens, B. (2002). *Trimbos/iMTA Questionnaire for Costs Associated with Psychiatric Illness (TiC-P)*. Rotterdam, The Netherlands: Instituut voor Medische Technology Assessment.

Hakkaart-van Roijen, L., Zwirs, B. W. C., Bouwmans, C., Tan, S. S., Schulpen, T. W. J., Vlasveld, L. & Buitelaar, J. K. (2007). Societal costs and quality of life of children suffering from attention deficient hyperactivity disorder (ADHD). *European Child & Adolescent Psychiatry*, *16*, 316-326. doi:10.1007/s00787-007-0603-6.

Haley, W. E., Levine, E. G., Brown, S. L., Berry, J. W. & Hughes, G. H. (1987). Psychological, social, and health consequences of caring for a relative with senile dementia. *Journal of the American Geriatrics Society*, *35*, 405-411.

Hoffmann, F. & Rodrigues, R. (2010). *Informal caregivers: who takes care of them?* Policy brief 4/2010. Vienna: European Centre.

Hong, S. (2010). Understanding patterns of service utilization among informal caregivers of community older adults. *The Gerontologist*, *50*, 87-99. doi:10.1093/geront/gnp105.

Hopps, M., Iadeluca, L., McDonald, M. & Makinson, G. T. (2017). The burden of family caregiving in the United States: work productivity, health care resource utilization, and mental health among employed adults. *Journal of Multidisciplinary Healthcare*, *10*, 437-444. doi:10.2147/JMDH.S135372.

Hulley, S. R., Cummings, W. S., Browner, D. G., Grady. & Newman, T. B. (2013). *Designing Clinical Research* (4th ed.). Philadelphia: Lippincott Williams & Wilkins.

Kolanowski, A. M., Fick, D., Waller, J. L. & Shea, D. (2004). Spouses of persons with dementia: their healthcare problems, utilization, and costs. *Research in Nursing & Health*, *27*, 296-306. doi:10.1002/ nur.20036.

Lee, M., Park, C., Matthews, A. K. & Hsieh, K. (2017). Differences in physical health, and health behaviors between family caregivers of children with and without disabilities. *Disability and Health Journal, 10*, 565-570. doi:10.1016/j.dhjo.2017.03.007.

Lee, S., Colditz, G. A., Berkman, L. F. & Kawachi, I. (2003). Caregiving and risk of coronary heart disease in U.S. women: a prospective study. *American Journal of Preventive Medicine*, *24*, 113-119. doi:10.1016/S0749-3797(02)00582-2.

Leggett, L. E., Khadaroo, R. G., Holroyd-Leduc, J., Lorenzetti, D. L., Hanson, H., Wagg, A. & Clement, F. (2016). Measuring resource utilization. A systematic review of validated self-reported questionnaires. *Medicine*, *95* (10), e2759. doi: 10.1097/ MD. 0000000000002759.

Longacre, M. L., Valdmanis, V. G., Handorf, E. A. & Fang, C. Y. (2017). Work impact and emotional stress among informal caregivers for older adults. *Journals of Gerontology: Social Sciences*, *72*, 522-531. doi:10.1093/geronb/gbw027.

Martindale-Adams, J., Nichols, L. O., Zuber, J., Burns, R. & Graney, M. J. (2016). Dementia caregivers' use of services for themselves. *The Gerontologist*, *56*, 1053-1061. doi:10.1093/geront/gnv121.

McQuaid, J. R., Stein, M. B., McCahill, M., Laffaye, C. & Ramel, W. (2000). Use of brief psychiatric screening measures in a primary care sample. *Depression & Anxiety*, *12*, 21–29. doi: 10.1002/1520-6394(2000)12:1<21::AID-DA3>3.0.CO;2-U.

Ministry of Health, Consumer Affairs and Social Welfare. (2018). *Encuesta Nacional de Salud España 2017 (presentación)* [*National Health Survey Spain (presentation)*]. Retrieved from: https://www.mscbs.gob.es/estad Estudios/estadisticas/encuestaNacional/encuesta2017.htm.

Musich, S., Wang, S. S., Kraemer, S., Hawkins, K. & Wicker, E. (2017). Caregivers for older adults: prevalence, characteristics, and health care utilization and expenditures. *Geriatric Nursing*, *38*, 9-16. doi:10.1016/j.gerinurse.2016.06.017.

National Alliance for Caregiving (NAC), Schulz, R. & Cook, T. (2011) was used set the unit cost per visit with a social worker. Caregiving costs.

Declining health in the Alzheimer's caregiver as dementia increases in the care recipient. Retrieved from https:// www.caregiving.org/pdf/ research/Alzheimers_Caregiving_Costs_Study_FINAL.pdf.

Perlick, D. A., Hohenstein, J. M., Clarkin, J. F., Kaczynski, R. & Rosenheck, R. A. (2005). Use of mental health and primary care services by caregivers of patients with bipolar disorder: a preliminary study. *Bipolar Disorder*, *7*, 126-135. doi:10.1111/j.1399-5618.2004.00172.x.

Pinquart, M. & Sörensen, S. (2003). Differences between caregivers and noncaregivers in psychological health and physical health: a meta-analysis. *Psychology and Aging*, *18*, 250-267. doi:10.1037/0882-7974.18.2.250.

Pruchno, R. A. & Potashnik, S. L. (1989). Caregiving spouses physical and mental health in perspective. *Journal of the American Geriatrics Society*, *37*, 697-705. doi:10.1111/j.1532-5415.1989.tb02230.x.

Rabarison, K. M., Bouldin, E. D., Bish, C. L., McGuire, L. C., Taylor, C. A. & Greenlund, K. J. (2018). The economic value of informal caregiving for persons with dementia: results from 38 States, the District of Columbia, and Puerto Rico, 2015 and 2016 BRFSS. *American Journal of Public Health*, *108*, 1370-1377. doi:10.2105/ AJPH.2018.304573.

Radloff, L. S. (1977). The CES-D Scale: A self-report depression scale for research in the general population. *Applied Psychological Measurement*, *1*, 385–401. doi: 10.1177/014662167700100306.

Reinhard, S. C., Feinberg, L. F., Choula, R. & Houser, A. (2015). *Valuing the invaluable: 2015 update. Insight on the Issues.* Retrieved from: https://www.aarp.org/content/dam/aarp/ppi/2015/valuing-the-invaluable-2015-update-new.pdf.

Salvador-Carulla, L., Bendeck, M., Fernández, A., Alberti, C., Sabes-Figuera, R., Molina, C. & Knapp, M. (2011). Costs of depression in Catalonia (Spain). *Journal of Affective Disorders*, *132*, 130-138. doi:10.1016/ j.jad.2011.02.019.

Schmitz, H. & Westphal, M. (2017). Informal care and long-term labor market outcomes. *Journal of Health Economics*, *56*, 1-18. doi:0.1016/ j.jhealeco.2017.09.002.

Schubert, C. C., Boustani, M., Callahan, C. M., Perkins, A. J., Hui, S. & Hendrie, H. C. (2008). Acute care utilization by dementia caregivers within urban primary care practices. *Journal of General Internal Medicine*, *23*, 1736-1740. doi: 10.1007/s11606-008-0711-0.

Sculpher, M., Pang, F., Manca, A., Drummond, M., Golder, S. & Urdahl, H. (2004). Generalisability in economic evaluation studies in healthcare: a review and case studies. *Health Technology Assessment*, *8*(49), iii-iv, 1-192. doi: 10.3310/hta8490.

Soeteman, D. I., Hakkaart-van Roijen, L., Verheul, R. & Busschbach, J. J. V. (2008). The economic burden of personality disorders in mental health care. *Journal of Clinical Psychiatry*, *69*, 256-265.

Stacey, A. F., Gill, T. K., Price, K. & Taylor, A. W. (2018). Differences in risk factors and chronic conditions between informal (family) carers and non-carers using a population-based cross-sectional survey in South Australia. *BMJ Open*, *8*. doi:10.1136/bmjopen-2017-020173.

Suehs, B. T., Shah, S. N., David, C. D., Alvir, J., Faison, W. E., Patel, N. & Bobula, J. (2014). Household members of person with Alzheimer's Disease: health conditions, healthcare use, and healthcare costs. *Journal of Geriatrics Society*, *62*, 435-441. doi:10.1111/jgs.12694.

Suzuki, K., Tamakoshi, K. & Sakakibara, H. (2016). Caregiving activities closely associated with the development of low-back pain among female family caregivers. *Journal of Clinical Nursing*, *25*, 2156-2167. doi:10.1111/jocn.13167.

Tan, S. S., Bouwmans, C. A. M., Rutten, F. F. H. & Hakkaart-van Roijen, L. (2012). Update of the Ducth Manual for costing in economic evaluations. *International Journal of Technology Assessment in Health Care*, *28*, 152-158. doi:10.1017/S0266462312000062.

Timman, R., Bouwmans, C., Busschbach, J. J. V. & Hakkaart-van Roijen, L. (2015). Development of the Treatment Inventory of Costs in Psychiatric Patients: TIC-P Mini and Midi. *Value in Health*, *18*, 994-999. doi:10.1016/j.jval.2015.07.006.

Toseland, R. W., McCallion, P., Gerber, T. & Banks, S. (2002). Predictors of health and human services use by persons with dementia and their family caregivers. *Social Science & Medicine*, *55*, 1255-1266. doi:10.1016/S0277-9536(01)00240-4.

Triantafillou, J., Naiditch, M., Repkova, K., Stiehr, K., Carretero, S., Emilsson, T. & Vlantoni, D. (2010). *Informal care in the long-term care system. European Overview paper.* Athens/Vienna: Interlinks. Retrieved from: https://www.euro.centre.org/downloads/detail/768.

van Houtven, C. H., Coe, N. B. & Skira, M. M. (2013). The effect of informal care on work and wages. *Journal of Health Economics*, *32*, 240-252. doi:10.1016/j.jhealeco.2012.10.006.

van Roijen, L., Essink-Bot, M. L., Koopmanschap, M. A., Bonsel, G. & Rutten, F. F. (1996). Labor and health status in economic evaluation of health care. The Health and Labor Questionnaire. *International Journal Technology Assessment in Health Care*, *12*, 405-415.

Vázquez, F. L., Blanco, V. & López, M. (2007). An adaptation of the Center for Epidemiologic Studies Depression Scale for use in non-psychiatric Spanish populations. *Psychiatry Research*, *149*, 247-252. doi:10.1016/ j.psychres.2006. 03.004.

Vilagut, G., Forero, C. G., Barbaglia, G. & Alonso, J. (2016). Screening for depression in the general population with the Center for Epidemiologic Studies Depression (CES-D): a systematic review with meta-analysis. *Plos One*, *11*, e0155431. doi: 10.1371/ journal.pone.0155431.

Vitaliano, P. P., Zhang, J. & Scanlan, J. M. (2003). Is caregiving hazardous to one's physical health? A meta-analysis. *Psychological Bulletin*, *129*, 946-972. doi:10.1037/0033-2909.129.6.946.

Wang, X. R., Robinson, K. & Carter-Harris, L. (2014). Prevalence of chronic illnesses and characteristics of chronically ill informal caregivers of persons with dementia. *Age and Ageing*, *43*, 137-141. doi:10.1093/ageing/aft142.

Zhu, C. W., Scarmeas, N., Ornstein, K., Albert, M., Brandt, J., Blacker, D. & Stern, Y. (2015). Healthcare use and cost in dementia caregivers: longitudinal results from the Predictors Caregiver Study. *Alzheimers & dementia: the Journal of the Alzheimer's Association*, *11*, 444-454. doi:10.1016/j.jalz.2013.12.018.

In: Caregiving
Editor: Stefano Eleuteri
ISBN: 978-1-53616-889-1

Chapter 4

SUPPORTING FAMILY CAREGIVERS OF OLDER ADULTS WITH HIP FRACTURE: THE ROLE OF EDUCATIONAL COURSES

Maria Eduarda Batista de Lima[1], Stefano Eleuteri[2,*] and Paolo Falaschi[1]

[1]Fragility Fracture Network, Education Committee, Rome, Italy
[2]Department of Psycology, Sapienza, University of Rome, Italy; Fragility Fracture Network, Education Committee, Rome Italy

ABSTRACT

Family caregivers' mental health is an important predictor of care recipients' institutionalization and a risk factor for care-recipient mortality. Caregiver burden and its associated stress negatively affect caregivers' perceived general physical and mental health and have been negatively correlated with the functional status of older adults family members after discharge following hip fracture surgery. The rehabilitation process is highly dependent on the quality of care provided by the family caregiver.

* Corresponding Author's Email: stefano.eleuteri@uniroma1.it.

Hip fracture is considered an acute event and often caregivers do not have enough time to develop the necessary skills and competencies to provide adequate care. The literature shows that interventions improving social support for family caregivers of older adults were found to effectively increase caregivers' confidence, coping ability and caregiver outcomes. The aim of this chapter is to discuss the importance of educational courses as support for family members of older adults who have suffered a hip fracture and present the results of a recent study we have carried out. The study was carried out on 398 caregivers of patients with hip fracture (mean age: 46.2, from 28 to 69 years). They were administered educational courses, consisting of 12 hours of frontal presentations and 30 hours of teledidactics. Each participant was given a socio-demographic questionnaire and, at the baseline and post-hoc, the Caregiver Burden Inventory (CBI) and a questionnaire to assess knowledge on hip fracture. A questionnaire was also administered to assess their satisfaction on the intervention. 52% of our sample was composed of family caregivers, 89% were females and 92% had Italian citizenship. The mean caregiving period was 28 months, the mean age of patients was 81.92 years (from 72 to 99), with 88.4% of the patients being females. At the baseline, the mean knowledge score was 12.3/21, while after the intervention 18.2/21. The mean CBI score was 28.85 at the baseline and 26.4 after the intervention. 95% of participants declared to have a high level of satisfaction regarding the course. These findings confirm the usefulness of caregiver educational courses in order to decrease caregiver burden and implement knowledge on hip fracture. Trainings and support group interventions are needed to better prepare family caregivers to make decisions, to feel confident to be part of the health care plan of their dependent relative and to know their rights; services provider should encourage the family carers to take care of their physical and psychological needs as well.

Keywords: caregiver's burden, hip fracture, educational support

INTRODUCTION

Caring for an older person living at home is an important issue to study since the ageing population is increasing and special attention should be given to the needs of the older person and their family caregivers, in order to increase their wellbeing and enable the older person to live at their homes as long as possible. Family caregivers require practical and psychological skills; therefore itis important to address the family carer's needs seriously (Bueckling, Struewer & Waldermann, 2014).

Depending on the family caregiver's circumstances, caring for relatives can be a joy or the care can be a source of anxiety. A person who needs a lot of help and care may cause a negative effect on the caregiver's quality of life, which can also affect the relationship between the caregiver and the caretaker (Neugaard, Andresen & McKune, 2008; Eleuteri, Bellanti & Falaschi, 2016).

The caregiving rehabilitation task associated with hip fracture fall, more often than not, to the lot of a member of the family (Young, Xiong & Pruzek, 2011). Studies have focused, in particular, on the concept of burden, defined as "burden of care", losing sight of the importance of assessing the positive aspects that characterize the state of health of an individual. Informal caregivers are an important resource for elderly patients suffering from hip fracture because they play a key role during their recovery. One important task is that of motivating the patients to adhere to their therapy programmes. Informal caregivers have to cope with physical, psychological and social stressors that affect their health conditions and quality of life negatively (Kristensen, 2011; Alarcón, González-Montalvo & Gotor, 2011; Fianco, Sartori & Negri, 2015).

Many caregivers assume the caregiver role with little or no preparation and have to learn to deal with several aspects of care in a very short time. Most often they have no professional skills in assistance procedure. In fact, more often than not, caregivers do not know what to expect during hip-fracture recovery. They face situations where they have to address various care-related tasks, such as arrangement of rehabilitation services and assistive devices. These situations become more stressful when caregivers have to juggle their own professional and family lives with their activities as carers; informal caregivers have been repeatedly acknowledged as a model of chronic stress, due to the high level of daily stress that caregivers experience (Eleuteri et al., 2018). The primary stressors experienced by informal caregivers are related to the severity of the ailment and the quantity of time devoted to assistance (Falaschi & Eleuteri, 2017).

When caregivers are monitored over considerably long periods of time, it becomes evident that family caregiving responsibilities do not end with institutionalisation of the disabled relative. Instead, this key transition appears to affect the type and intensity of help provided. Unlike earlier studies that treated institutionalisation as an 'endpoint' in family caregiving, recent research has emphasised the continued involvement of relatives in care and the effects of nursing-home admission upon the stress and mental health of family members (McCullagh, Brigstocke & Donaldson, 2005).

There is a lack of literature addressing family caregiving for frail elderly people and its consequence on the life quality of family caregivers. The subjective responses of individuals to the environments in which they live play an important role in maintaining the status of their care recipients. High levels of depressive symptoms and low levels of life satisfaction in caregivers may also be associated with the low quality of the care provided to their frail care-recipients and even with maltreatment of the older adult (Morimoto, Schreiner & Asano, 2003). Caregiver burden and its associated stress impact negatively upon caregivers' perceived general physical and mental health and have been negatively correlated with the functional status of elderly family members 1 month after discharge following hip fracture surgery (Lin & Lu, 2005; Shyu, Chen & Liang, 2012; Liu, Yang & Cheng, 2015).

Researches show that family caregivers mostly need support and information. The issues most often mentioned by the family caregiver in a study were the need for advice in complicated situations (61%) and the need for information about medication and psychiatry (60%) (Reinhard, Given & Petlick, 2008).

Studies show that, in order for the family carer to reduce their own distress, it is required to have both skills and knowledge to provide care (Given, Given & Stommel, 1999; National Alliance for Caregiving, 2004).

According to Clyburn,Stones, and Hadjistavropoulos (2000), many family carers say that they do not receive enough guidance from providers on how to assume the carer's role, that they do not have the skills and information necessary to provide care and do not know where to access it and therefore they feel unprepared to care for a person with chronic illness that can lead to a problematic situation since the family carers wellbeing is often strongly connected to their care situation, how it is interpreted, as a burden or not.

REVIEW

Supporting Caregivers by the Empowerment Concept

The philosophical concepts of empowerment can be traced from Latin America and Paulo Freire and his 'Pedagogy of the Oppressed' to others philosophers such as Sartre.

The idea behind the empowerment concept is that it is possible to help people to cope and feel better through dialogue and reflection between the professional and the client who needs, or between the family carer and the caretaker. According to Freire, within an empowerment strategy, the professional should encourage the person to expose their own weakness and resources when facing illness and other limitations in order to reflect to gether on the meaning of the illness and to promote the client's choice to act and cope.

Although Freire's theory on consciousness-raising among under-privileged groups (Schulz & Sherwood, 2008; Thomas, 2017) was not in relation to illness, the idea is to say that by encouraging the clients to think about their situations is a way to make the power come from the clients and for changes to happen, that empowerment highlights client's competences, and that there are many different solutions to one problem (Hage & Lorensen, 2005).

According to Adams (2008), empowerment is the ability of individuals or groups to be in charge of the situation and accomplish their own goals. It is the process by which, individually or collectively, people are able to increase the quality of their lives and help themselves. The provision of education, resources and self awareness is seeing as an empowerment process, giving great power to the clients.

One important association with empowerment is democracy, where individual's choice and freedom are vital. However, empowerment can have different meanings for different people; it can be a feeling of being valued and recognized; to get feedback that there are doing a significant job; to have the necessary resources; feeling of freedom; to have the proper caring skills and so on. Empowerment accurately means "become powerful" in the Dictionary of Social Work and it is linked with self help,that is defined as ways that people help themselves (Adams, 2008).

Research shows that, in order to empower a person, it is necessary to have a holistic approach, to consider all aspects of the person's needs, such as social, spiritual, emotional and physical ones.Simply inviting a person to participate will not cause empowerment, therefore it is important to have the person's private experiences and thoughts being in harmony with what they do. The empowerment process is a continuous interaction involving empowering practice and critical reflections. However, practitioners need to become empowered themselves first, before empowering others, since a person needs competence and motivation in order to empower others (Adams, 2008). Empowerment of family carers can be achieved in many ways and it is based on the family members' situations and experiences that it is possible to define their own needs.

One way to empower a person is by preventing exhaustion and diminishing stressful factors. Another form of empowerment is through counseling, to empower the carer to discover their own needs, to evaluate the cause of their problems for themselves and find their own strategies (Lloyd & Carson, 2005).

In his study, Carr (2003) states that the level of participation by caregivers (mainly family members) in empowerment groups is still low. This is due to the fact that assistance activities take time and generate tiredness and they often feel discouraged or unwilling to participate. Empowerment of family carers can be achieved in different ways because there are a number of issues to consider that can decrease the family carer's load and can promote empowerment, such as to provide enough information about care, help the family carers to recognize their own needs, provide time for family carers' recreation, encourage family carers to keep in touch with friends and others with similar experiences and finally provide financial support (Clarke, 2001).

Caregiver's life is made up of different aspects

that affect their wellbeing and empowerment. The family carer should analyze each aspect and conclude which one is taking them down, where they need help and actively start the changes. The family carer empowerment can be jeopardized after a family member's health deteriorates, because such a large part of the family carer's days is devoted to the caretaker, consuming a lot of energy and often the situation starts to dominate their ownidentity (Bickman & Heflinger, 1998).

In situations whereby the caregiving context changes, the carer role identity in relation to the cared person also changes and this can cause distress for some. For example, when the family carer realizes that his/her duties are extending from the initial role such as paying bills, shopping to more personal needs such as personal grooming, it can cause for some family carers a lot of discomfort which can lead the family carer to leave his/her role and place the cared person in a nursing home for example. It is important to notice that not every family caregiver goes through the same process and distress and burden are not linear (Montgomery & Kosloski, 2012).

To decrease family carers feeling of burden and help them to keep a role that they would like to have, it is very important to provide enough information and education training . Family carers have to recognize their own needs and emotions and set limitations in order to support their own wellbeing by keeping a separate identity. It is particularly important to create and offer the family carers support services and their own peer support forums where caregivers can exchange experiences and get comfort (Lloyd & Carson, 2005).

Often when asking a family carer, "How are you doing?" they respond with reference to the condition of the caretaker. It is usually difficult for the family carer to think that while supporting the caretaker does not have to mean neglecting their own feelings and needs.

Sometimes it takes a long time before the family carer starts to see their real self again, without feeling guilt and the main issue in order to empower the family carer is to recreate the one's self and set the limitations for how much one is able to do. After that, the family carer can set goals and recognize their needs (Bickman & Heflinger, 1998).

There are different ways in order to empower the family carer and help the person to overcome difficulties; however an overview of this person life is needed. Research shows that seldom the family carer thinks of themselves first; however, the quality of life of the family carer is strongly related to the family carer's coping skills and wellbeing (Clarke, 2001).

When developing an education training in order to empower the family carer, it is first needed an analysis of the family carer's coping skills, an overview of the family carer's daily routine, interests, sleep routines and so on (Lloyd & Carson, 2005).

Educational Trainings for Caregivers

The scientific literature shows that educational training programmes are a vehicle to empower the family carer; improving family carer's burden and depression: increasing family carer's capacity to better control emotional experiences when facing problematic situations; enhancing skills for effective problem solving; increasing family care's knowledge about different diseases and treatment; providing guidance and psychological support; increasing family carer's knowledge about their rights and supportservices offered for family carers (Clarke, 2001; Stolz, 2004; Campbell, 2004).

However, an analysis of how and if an educational training programme has been able to empower family carers by providing information showed that the training increased family carer's knowledge about their rights and support services available to the family carers but did not increase family carer's self-esteem, perceived control and competence.

Results showed that the short duration of the training which was a one day workshop affected the outcomes, therefore the course should be of a longer duration, providing opportunity for family carers to practice their skills at home and a follow-up should occur over a longer period than 2 weeks (Clarke, 2001). Empowerment is a constant process that can be achieved by external interference whereby family carers become able to express their needs and the service provider should meet those needs by not only including the family carer in the decision making related to the care and by increasing family carer's knowledge but by enhancing individual self-efficacy and competence, meeting the family carers's psychological needs with the provision of a several weeks course including learning activities in order for family carers to put in practice their new skills (Sakanashi & Fujita, 2017).

A longitudinal study analyzing the impact of a nurse-led support and educational programme for spouses, caring for a family member that had a stroke aimed to provide opportunity for spouses to ask questions and exchange experiences with others family carers in similar situation, with the goal to improve the family carers knowledge about stroke. Results showed that participants that attended the programme for 5-6 times during six months had an increase of well-being and quality of life. However it might also be important to include in the programme coping strategies with an empowerment approach (Larson, 2005).

According to a systematic literature review on support for family carers (Stoltz, Uden & Willman, 2004), it was found that depending on the medical diagnosis of the person being cared can influence family carers's need for support.

The findings of the systematic literature review were divided in different categories, including the need of support, supportive interven-tions, experiences of family caregiving and ethnicity.

Results showed that family carers, dealing with the caregiving demand, with more problem solving approach, rather than emotional focused coping skills, were less burdened. In addition, results showed that family carers express needs to learn about medication and depression; to share their experiences in peer groups and family carers they expressed their wish to have more social contacts, learn ways to cope with their feelings, information and education. In addition, family carers expressed fear of isolation and for the caretaker safety.

A study about family carer empowerment resulted in the development of a variety of leaflets based on the family carer's needs and the family carers were involved in the leaflet's development process. Results of the research showed that family carers recognized that one of the causes for their stress is the feeling of anger, guilt and loss that their caretakers are suffering from their condition. Therefore it is important that family carers can get assistance in how to support the caretaker as well. The leaflets were 'carer friendly', easy to access and to understand. The leaflets included agencies offering support to the family caregivers, mental health services; the most used terminologies by professionals; early warning signs of diseases and treatments; what to do in emergency situations; about the law; how to recognize stress signs and how to cope (Llyod & Carson, 2005).

Another study that have similar finding is the one of Sinnakaruppan, Downey and Morrison (2005), which proposes that empower the family carer can be done with the use of handouts with basic information about memory problems; ways to cope; memory aids; how to encourage the patient and the family carer.

Another approach of educational/support training for family carers is thought behavioral family therapy (BFT). Families selected to participate had at least one family member suffering from a mental illness. Results of the qualitative study, evaluating experiences of families that received BFT, showed that family carers felt empowered to ask for help.

A qualitative research describes or explores the experience of a certain phenomenon rather than generalize conclusion to a large population (Campbell, 2004). In addition, result showed empowerment of the families involved. The majority of families reported that BFT increased communication among family members, since BFT encourage participants to communicate in an effective way; decreasing stress and feeling of isolation, and new coping skills were acquired.(Campbell, 2004).

Another important aspect researched was the impact that mental health problems can cause in terms of quality of life for both the family carer and the caretaker with intellectual disabilities. A guide was developed to support family carers. Result showed that increasing family carer's consciousness of the related issues can be a way to promote mental health and increase family carers wellbeing since it is likewise important for the family caregiever to know how to keep their own mental health. Information and knowledge about treatments, illness and services and presenting this information in an easy way can be helpful for the family carer's and caretaker's empowerment (Gratsa, 2007).

The overall analysis of the literature review concerning supporting services in terms of educational training and information services for family carers are very beneficial, improving the family carers' well-being and promoting the family carer empowerment (Rodgers, Atkinson & Bond, 1999; Funk, Stajduhar, Giesbrecht, Cloutier, Williams & Wolse, 2019).

There are different ways to empower family caregivers through educational trainings and information services. However these services should provide opportunity for family carers to express their needs, it should include ways to help the carer to better control their emotions and to increase coping/problem solving skills. In addition, information about family caregiver's rights and support services offered to the family carer should be provided. It's very important that educational trainings and information services are well planned in order to increase the family carers self confidence by providing the right kind of skills and knowledge, for example about medication and depression. Family carers also could be empowered by enhancing their competence and self-esteem, throuth verbalization of their psychological needs. Results show that family carers can get empowered by sharing their experiences with others in similar situations, therefore open communication among participants in an educational training should be encouraged to decrease stress and feelings of isolation among family carers. Furthermore result showed that coping strategies with an empowerment approach should be included in the programmes.

Additionally, results showed that educational trainings should be of a longer duration than one day, that better outcomes were achieved with courses that last for 5-6 times sincc longer courses provide more opportunities for family carers to practice their new skills at home and that a follow up should occur over longer period than two weeks.

The analysis of the literature review related to the support services in terms of provision of information showed that family carers can be empowered with the use of hand outs with basic information about memory problems, knowledge about treatments, illness and services available for the family carer. However that the information should be easy to access and interpret as well as very helpful for the family carer's and caretaker's empowerment. Therefore educational training should be combined with the provision of handouts and leaflets specially developed for family caregivers (Nahm, Resnick & Orwig, 2010; Bunn, Lynch, Goodman, Sharpe, Walshe, Preston & Froggatt, 2018).

Approaching the Family Carer during Educational Training Using Technology

There are many countries in Europe investing in gerontechnology, developing assistive devices that benefit the daily tasks of the family carers, including the provision of a diverse number of different security devices, such as night alarms, security telephone, locomotion detection and so on. In addition to assistive devices, new technologies are used in order to provide education training and information for family carers by telematics (Mestheneos & Triantafillou, 2005).

Telematics can be defined as the application of information and communications technologies and services; a telematics application is a system or a service meeting user needs (Chambers & Connor, 2002).

Gerontechnology according Graafmas (1992) describes that the main purpose of gerontechnology is to support the older adult in 5 different ways: compensation, prevention, enhancement, care support and research. This definition says that gerontechnology can support the family carers in a variety of ways, enhancing their quality of life providing more time and less physical effort for the family carers, automatically reducing the stress and enhancing life satisfaction.

Graafmas says that the research and development of technological products and techniques, are based on the research of the human ageing and the aim is to create a better working and living environment, doing the needed adjustments in order to provide better quality of life for the older person.

There are a lot of new innovations considering gerontechonolgy at the moment and the numbers are increasing all the time. Technological innovations are of a great help for the older person and their family caregivers, enabling the older persons to stay at their homes in a safer environments. There are a number of devices that can help with daily and instrumental activities, such as eating device, locomotion devices, security devices such as, cooker, watch informing the person when the food is ready, security carpets and floors that detect movements, night alarms that are developed to wake the family caregiver when the caretaker moves from the bed and so on (Bouman, 1998).

The use of technology has numerous benefits it can be used to educate and engage family caregivers, can provide regular monitoring, such as alerting the client when it's time to take his/her medication, can increases client's safety with the assistance of remote motions that can be placed around the home detecting unusual movements and also has the potential to decrease the number of hours of personal assistance a cared person needs, it can help people that lives in rural area to reach health care providers, it can improve or maintain disable individuals functional capacities and increase safety on ADLs (Activities of Daily Living) and IADLs (Instrumental Activity of Daily Living) tasks and so on.

Assistance device can be very helpful for family caregivers and for the caretaker, improving outcomes and preventing increasing levels of stress faced by the family caregiver, as long as it is easy to learn how to use it, however necessary training should be offered to the family caregivers to master the new technology not causing more stress (Micera, Bonato & Tamura, 2008).

The problem is that technology can have a high cost, although it may significantly improve the clients' outcomes (Raphael & Cornwell, 2008).

Researchers studied the benefits of provision of information and communication technology for older people and their family caregivers in Sweden as a support service for older adults and their family caregivers. This study is part of bigger project investigating the impact of a technology-based service known as ACTION (Assisting Carers using Telematics Interventions to meet Older Person's Needs) a service that empowers older people and their family caregivers by providing information that can help them to make decisions concerning their caring situations. The Swedish ACTION services increased work satisfaction among professional staff and the municipalities involved in the project decided to implement ACTION as a continuous support services for family caregivers. The conclusion was that this kind of support service is cost effective, diminishing demand on staff and benefiting the users (Magnusson & Hanson, 2005).

Considering the different services purposes, it's hard to compare the benefits of ACTION with other services such as nursing home or home help. ACTION services can be increased in the future for example by virtual home visit by doctors, alarm systems can be installed and monitor health status at a good price as the families using ACTION already have the necessary equipments such as Internet access, broadband, computer and videophone. Overall this study result showed that the family carers felts more independent and secure to carry their caring tasks and felt less isolated (Magnusson & Hanson, 2005).

Furthermore other researches investigate how useful it is a multimedia software application, consisted of an information package planned to offer family members caring for the elderly or disabled with information, guidance, psychological support, including relaxation and other ways of coping. The multimedia software was evaluated in order to find out if the family carer coping capacity could increase by providing family carers with coping methods, advice, and promotion of psychological health. An evaluation questionnaire was used to improve and develop the content and usability of the multimedia software application. Results showed that a way to empower the family carer is by increasing family carer's coping skills, that family carer's need emotional support, to better cope with the new role. In addition result showed that the most of the users found the software to be educational and practical, therefore the author concluded that those who are caring for a older person and disabled at home can get support and information through the software application (Chambers & Coonor, 2002).

A pilot study of how information and communication technology (ICT) may contribute to health promotion among elderly spousal carers in Norway showed that the use of ICT by providing information about caring, coping skills, illness was beneficial to the family carers. Results showed that family carer's stress level reduced and their social network increased, family carers reported to be better prepared to deal with their spouses' illness, which automatically affect positively their mood and self confidence, resulting in empowerment. The use of information and communication technology (ICT) resulting in the family carer empowerment, increased family care's confidence and well-being, however this study also had limitations such as that it was not randomized controlled study and the intervention group was small. Result indicates that the use of ICT can benefit family carers providing care for a spouse with dementia or stroke. However it was difficult to interpret the contradictory result related to stress level and mental wellbeing but the reason for this could be related to the care taker health deterioration and the need of more help, in addition to the family carer health status. Overall the analyzed focus group data showed that family carers were better prepares to deal with their spouse's illness by getting ICT information, education and support. This pilot study services was included as part of the regular healthcare service in the participating municipalities because of the positive results. Therefore ICT has the potential to help with health promotion among family carers by providing information, education and support (Torp, 2008).

Therefore technology development is an important vehicle to increase or maintain the ability of older people to remain more independent at home, which can automatically facilitate the family carer's life in many ways, promoting their well-being and increasing quality of life (Torp & Hanson, 2008).

Our Research

Introduction

Caregivers are an important resource for older adults with hip fracture, mainly if they are a family member, because they play a key role in their recovery process. Moreover, they have the important task of motivating the patients to join the therapy programme (Zarit, Stephens & Townsend, 1998). Caregivers often neglect their own needs and personal lives due to their assistance tasks; this may also prove to be a source of stress negatively affecting the caregiver's and patient's quality of life (Roth, Mittleman & Clay, 2005). With the aims of enhancing the figure and role of the caregiver; of empowering family carers, by improving their knowledge, self-confidence, coping skills, social network and well-being; of decreasing caregiver burden and implementing knowledge on hip fracture; of encouraging the practice of health education, we have built a multidisciplinary educational course to support caregivers of patients with hip fracture. We also evaluated the effects of the course on the level of knowledge on the fracture and on the burden level of caregivers.

METHODS

Sample and Procedures

The study was carried-out on 398 caregivers of patients with hip fracture in different Italian regions. They were administered educational courses, consisting of 12 hours of frontal presentations and 30 hours of teledidactics.

Each participant was given a socio-demographic questionnaire and, at the baseline and post-hoc, the Caregiver Burden Inventory (CBI) and a questionnaire to assess knowledge on hip fracture. A questionnaire was also administered to assess their satisfaction on the intervention.

The Caregiver Burden Inventory (CBI)

The Multidimensional Caregiver Burden Inventory (CBI) 42 is a 24-item Likert-format scale (0-4) that measures 5 dimensions of the caregiver burden: time- dependence, developmental, physical, social, and emotional burden. The time-dependence burden emanates from the time demands and restrictions that caregiving can impose on caregivers, whereas the developmental burden describes the caregivers' feelings of being 'offtime' in their development with respect to their peers. The physical burden refers to the strain associated with demands on caregivers' physical health, strength, and energy. The social burden refers to 'caregivers' negative feelings toward their care recipients, which may also result from the patient's unpredictable and often bizarre behaviour.

The CBI comprises 24 closed questions. There are five items in each dimension except for physical burden, which has four. Each item is attributed a score between 0 (not at all descriptive) and 4 (very descriptive), where higher scores indicate greater caregiver burden; there are no cut-off points for classifying burden (Novak & Guest, 1989).

Increasing numbers of studies have examined the caregiver-burden phenomenon, the lack of support given to caregivers and intervention focused on relieving the caregiver burden; this increase is probably due, in part, to greater evidence that caregiver burden is a determining factor of caregivers' Quality of Life (QoL) (Jonsson, Lindgren & Hallstrom, 2005). Social support has been associated with a diminution of caregiver burden (Lin & Lu, 2007). High care-demand levels may affect multiple aspects of caregivers' lives, including their free time, social life, emotional and physical health, as well as their personal development. These subjectively defined stressors are also called caregiver burden. Perceived caregiver burden may affect their self-esteem, sense of competency as caregivers and the degree of growth due to dealing with caregiving challenges, adversely (Pearlin, Mullan & Semple, 1990; Carretero, Garcés & Ródenas, 2009).

Socio-Demographic Questionnaire

In the socio-demographic questionnaire information about caregiver's age and degree of of kinship was found. Also, information about caregiver's citizenship, type of constraint with the assisted (family or family assistant), caregiving period, patient's gender and age.

Questionnaire to Assess Knowledge on Hip Fracture

The questionnaire was composed of 21 questions, with true and false statements. The questionnaire contained theoretical and practical aspects in hip fracture. The questionnaire was administered at the beginning and at the end of the course.

Course Evaluation Questionnaire

This survey evaluated the opinion of caregivers regarding organizational efficiency; congruence of content; exhibition clarity; structural quality and suggestions.

Statistics

Data collection was transferred to the software Epi Info™ and was analyzed by the same. Epi Info™ is a public domain suite of interoperable software tools designed for the global community of public health practitioners and researchers. It provides for easy data entry form and database construction, a customized data entry experience, and data analyses with epidemiologic statistics, maps, and graphs for public health professionals who may lack an information technology background.

RESULTS

During the frontal presentations, the meetings were led by medical specialists (orthogeriatricians), nurses and psychologists. All professionals guaranteed the space for verbalizing any doubts or experiences experienced by caregivers.

The topics of the frontal presentations have been grouped into modules (Table 1) and exposed to caregivers through slides, with an easy to understand and fluent language. In the e-learning platform, the caregivers were able to find many in-depth materials, such illustrative videos integrating each module; book chapters, web links etc. A communication channel between caregivers and educators was created within the platform to ensure listening, course accompaniment and the resolution of doubts.

The e-learning platform used was Moodle of Sapienza University of Rome.

Sociodemographic characteristics of the sample are presented on Table 2. 52% of our sample was composed of family caregivers, 89% were females and 92% had Italian citizenship. The mean caregiving period was 28 months, the mean age of patients was 81.92 years (from 72 to 99), with 88.4% of the patients being females.

Table 1. Modules of "Educational course for caregivers of patients with hip fracture"

Module 1	Osteoporosis as cause of fragility fracture
Module 2	Frailty and sarcopenia
Module 3	Secondary prevention: falls, adherence of anti-osteoporosis treatment and importance of calcium and vitamin D supplementation
Module 4	Nutrition and hydration
Module 5	Notions of hygiene
Module 6	Techniques of mobilisation
Module 7	Skin care and injury prevention
Module 8	Mobility and exercises
Module 9	Supporting fracture patients with cognitive impairment
Module 10	Family carers' psychological needs
Module 11	Effective communication with the fractured patient
Module 12	The management of stress
Module 13	Social networks resource

Table 2. Sociodemographic characteristics of caregivers

n = 328 caregivers
Family caregivers: 52% (mainly daughters and granddaughters) Family assistants: 35% Healthcare Professionals: 7% Not specified: 6%
Caregiver's gender: 89% females
Caregiver's mean age: 46,22 years old (from 28 to 69 years old)
Citizenship: 92% Italian
Mean caregiving period: 28 months
Mean age of patients: 81,92 years old (from 72 to 99 years old)
Patient's gender: 88,4% female

At the baseline, the mean knowledge assessment score was 12.3/21, while after the intervention was 18.2/21.

The mean CBI score was 28.85 at the baseline and 26.4 after the intervention.

95% of participants declared to have a high level of satisfaction regarding the course and also have stated that they were more confident in managing their family members post a hip fracture.

Based on the first results of the knowledge test on hip fractures, we tried to personalize the contents of the course (frontal and e-learning) to give answers aimed at the doubts and needs of caregivers. We have also noted different needs between family caregivers and non-family members. While family caregivers presented doubts regarding the emotional sphere of the relationship with the fractured patient (e.g., how to communicate better with the patient), non-family caregivers presented doubts concerning the technical sphere of the relationship (e.g., how to mobilize the patient in bed, how to perform proper patient hygiene).

DISCUSSION

During our research we noted that the scientific literature presents few articles concerning the educational support to caregivers of people with hip fractures. Common are studies on the experiences of support to caregivers of patients with other kind of clinical condition, such as, cancer, stroke, Alzheimer and heart failure.

The increased risk of burnout identified among informal caregivers is closely related to their perceived level of burden, defined as a multidimensional response to negative appraisals and perceived stress (Falaschi & Eleuteri, 2017). Joint assessment of the burden and well-being dimensions, that coexist in caregivers' experiences, allows for the identification of personal and relational resources that may be usefully included in interventions addressed to caregivers (Fianco, Sartori & Negri, 2015; Falaschi, Eleuteri & Mitroi, 2015). In a recent preliminary study, we also found a correlation between patients' psychological well-being and caregivers' burdens (Fianco, Sartori & Negri, 2015).

This denotes the importance of carrying out other studies involving the caregivers of patients with hip fracture and to continue our research. In the light of the data obtained, our goal is to flood intervention times and perform a follow-up to verify the outcomes of the course on caregivers after 6 and 12 months. It also makes part of our objectives to include eventual outcomes of the course even on fractured patients (the caretakers), correlating the results obtained with a control group.

The reduction of the scores of burden and the increase in the average knowledge assessment score obtained after the course agrees with the literature. The analysis of the literature review related to the support services in terms of provision of information showed that family carers can be empowered with the use of hand outs with basic information about memory problems, knowledge about treatments, illness and services available for the family carer (Reinhard, 1994; Barg, Pasacreta & Nuamah, 1998; Teri, McCurry & Logsdon, 2005).

Furthermore, the results of the analysis of the literature review related to the use of ICT (information and communication technology) were very positive, that those who are caring for the older people and disabled at home can get support and information through software applications. Most of the users found the software to be educational and practical. Family carers reported an increase in their coping skills, reduction in their stress level and an increase of their social network, family carers reported to be better prepared to deal with their caretaker illness, among other things (Torp, 2007: Reinhard, Given & Petlick, 2008).

The National Institute for Health and Care Excellence (NICE) guideline on the management of hip fracture highlights the requirement for a multidisciplinary team in the care of patients with this condition and their caregivers. There is also an emphasis on providing patient-centred and continuous care across all disciplines and organisational boundaries; as such patients often cross specialties. Good communication is essential, and it should be supported by evidence-based information, to allow patients and their carers, where appropriate, to reach informed decisions about their care (NICE, 2011).

During our course the multidisciplinary aspect has been enhanced. The meetings were conducted mostly by orthogeriaters, nurses and psychologists. This aspect, together with the possibility of telephone and e-mail contact in case of doubts or any difficulties, have contributed to the high level of satisfaction of the course by the caregivers.

Our caregiver sample demonstrates the anthropological phenomenon of feminization of care.

All over the world, women are the predominant providers of informal care for family members with chronic medical conditions or disabilities, including the elderly and adults with mental illnesses. It has been suggested that there are several societal and cultural demands on women to adopt the role of a family-caregiver. Stress-coping theories propose that women are more likely to be exposed to caregiving stressors, and are likely to perceive, report and cope with these stressors differently from men. Many studies, which have examined gender differences among family-caregivers of people with mental illnesses, have concluded that women spend more time in providing care and carry out personal-care tasks more often than men (Wallsten SS, 2000; Adams, Aranda, Kemp & Takagi, 2002; Yeates, 2012).

These studies have also found that women experience greater mental and physical strain, greater caregiver-burden, and higher levels of psychological distress while providing care. However, almost an equal number of studies have not found any differences between men and women on these aspects. This has led to the view that though there may be certain differences between male and female caregivers, most of these are small in magnitude and of doubtful clinical significance. Accordingly, caregiver-gender is thought to explain only a minor proportion of the variance in negative caregiving outcomes. With changing demographics and social norms men are increasingly assuming roles as caregivers. However, the experience of men while providing care has not been explored adequately. The impact of gender on caregiving outcomes may be mediated by several other variables including patient-related factors, socio-demographic variables, and effects of kinship status, culture and ethnicity, but these have seldom been considered in the research on gender differences. Finally, it is apparent that methodological variations in samples, designs and assessments between studies contribute a great deal to the observed gender differences (De Regt, 2011).

Post-hip fracture life involves adapting the patient and his or her family to a new lifestyle and habits. Also involves taking charge that does not end with the patient's discharge and his return home. The reduction or the loss of the patient's autonomy involves the commitment of several hours of care by the caregiver. According to the International Osteoporosis Foundation (IOF), during the first year after a fracture, the hours of care provided by relatives vary greatly by fracture type: the more serious the fracture, the more support is needed.

The main period of care presented by our sample was 28 months. Parallel to the concern about the recovery of the acute event, there is also surveillance to avoid a secondary event and a new fracturing. Another aspect not to be underestimated is the adherence to drug therapy (mainly anti-osteoporotic therapy), the intake of calcium and vitamin D, as secondary prevention.

These important aspects, on which caregivers have a fundamental role and that increase even more the hours of care have, been approached during the course.

In front of the complexity that an event like a hip fracture can have on the patient's-caregiver's life, our study has demonstrated the importance of the educational support on decreasing burden and implement knowledge on hip fracture. Trainings and support group interventions are needed to better prepare family caregivers to make decisions, to feel confident to be part of the health care plan of their dependent relative, to know their rights and services provider should encourage the family carers to take care of their physical and psychological needs as well. Taking care of the patient-caregivers system from an educational and psychological point of view, from a clinical and education perspective will increase patients' quality of life and their full recovery possibilities.

REFERENCES

Adams, B., Aranda, M. P., Kemp, B., & Takagi, K. (2002). *Journal of Clinical Geropsychology*, *8*(4), 279–301. doi: 10.1023/a:1019627323558.

Adams, R. (2008). *Empowerment, participation and social work*. Basingstoke: Palgrave Macmillan, ISBN 978-0-230-01999-7.

Alarcón, T., González-Montalvo, J. I., Gotor, P., Madero, R., & Otero, A. (2010). Activities of daily living after hip fracture: profile and rate of recovery during 2 years of follow-up. *Osteoporosis International*, *22*(5), 1609–1613. doi: 10.1007/s00198-010-1314-2.

Barg, F. K., Pasacreta, J. V., Nuamah, I. F., Robinson, K. D., Angeletti, K., Yasko, J. M., & Mccorkle, R. (1998). A Description of a Psychoeducational Intervention for Family Caregivers of Cancer Patients. *Journal of Family Nursing*, *4*(4), 394–413. doi: 10.1177/107484079800400406.

Bickman, L., Heflinger, C. A., Northrup, D., Sonnichsen, S., & Schilling, S. (1998). Long Term Outcomes to Family Caregiver Empowerment. *Journal of Child and Family Studies*, *7*(3), 269–282. doi: 10.1023/a:1022937327049.

Bouman H. in Graafmans, J. (1998). *Gerontechnology a sustainable investment in the future*. Amsterdam: IOS Press.

Buecking, B., Struewer, J., Waldermann, A., Horstmann, K., Schubert, N., Balzer-Geldsetzer, M., … Bliemel, C. (2013). What determines health-related quality of life in hip fracture patients at the end of acute care?—a prospective observational study. *Osteoporosis International*, *25*(2), 475–484. doi: 10.1007/s00198-013-2415-5.

Bunn, F., Lynch, J., Goodman, C., Sharpe, R., Walshe, C., Preston, N., & Froggatt, K. (2018). Improving living and dying for people with advanced dementia living in care homes: a realist review of Namaste Care and other multisensory interventions. *BMC geriatrics*, *18*(1), 303. doi:10.1186/s12877-018-0995-9.

Campbell, A. S. (2004). How was it for you? Families experiences of receiving Behavioural Family Therapy. *Journal of Psychiatric and*

Mental Health Nursing, *11*(3), 261–267. doi: 10.1111/j.1365-2850.2003.00696.x.

Carretero, S., Garcés, J., Ródenas, F., & Sanjosé, V. (2009). The informal caregivers burden of dependent people: Theory and empirical review. *Archives of Gerontology and Geriatrics*, *49*(1), 74–79. doi: 10.1016/j.archger.2008.05.004.

Carr, E. S. (2003). Rethinking Empowerment Theory Using a Feminist Lens: The Importance of Process. *Affilia*, *18*(1), 8–20. doi: 10.1177/0886109902239092.

Chambers, M., & Connor, S. L. (2002). User-friendly technology to help family carers cope. *Journal of Advanced Nursing*, *40*(5), 568–577. doi: 10.1046/j.1365-2648.2002.02415.x.

Clarke, N. (2001). Training as a vehicle to empower carers in the community: more than a question of information sharing. *Health and Social Care in the Community*, *9*(2), 79–88. doi: 10.1046/j.1365-2524.2001.00284.x.

Clyburn, L., Stones, M., & Hadjistavropoulos, T. (2000). Predicting caregiver burden and depression in Alzheimers disease. *The Journals of Gerontology Series B: Psychological Sciences and Social Sciences*, *55*(1). doi: 10.1093/geronb/55.1.s2.

Creber, R. M. M., Hickey, K. T., & Maurer, M. S. (2016). Gerontechnologies for Older Patients with Heart Failure: What is the Role of Smartphones, Tablets, and Remote Monitoring Devices in Improving Symptom Monitoring and Self-Care Management? *Current Cardiovascular Risk Reports*, *10*(10). doi: 10.1007/s12170-016-0511-8.

Eleuteri, S., Bellanti, G. & Falaschi, P. (2016). Hip fracture: preliminary results supporting significant correlations between the psychological wellbeing of patients and their relative caregivers, *Journal of Gerontology & Geriatrics*, 64:104-111.

Eleuteri, S., Norton, M. C., Livi, F., Grano, C., Lucidi, F., Violani, C., … Lombardo, C. (2018) Sleep quality as predictor of BMI in non-depressed caregivers of people with dementia, *Eating and Weight Disorders*, 23(5), 553-560. doi: 10.1007/s40519-018-0560-8.

Epi Info™. (2018, November 16). Retrieved from https://www.cdc.gov/epiinfo/index.html.

Falaschi, P., Eleuteri, S., & Mitroi, C. (2015). Hip fracture: relation between patient's and caregiver's psychological wellbeing. In: *Abstracts of the 4th Fragility Fracture Network Congress*, Rotterdam, Netherlands, 3-5 September 2015:75-6.

Falaschi, P., & Eleuteri, S. (2016). The Psychological Health of Patients and Their Caregivers. *Practical Issues in Geriatrics Orthogeriatrics*, 201–211. doi: 10.1007/978-3-319-43249-6_14.

Fianco, A., Sartori, R. D., Negri, L., Lorini, S., Valle, G., & Fave, A. D. (2015). The relationship between burden and well-being among caregivers of Italian people diagnosed with severe neuromotor and cognitive disorders. *Research in Developmental Disabilities*, *39*, 43–54. doi: 10.1016/j.ridd.2015.01.006.

Funk, L. M., Stajduhar, K. I., Giesbrecht, M., Cloutier, D., Williams, A., & Wolse, F. (2019). Applying the concept of structural empowerment to interactions between families and home-care nurses. *Nursing Inquiry*. doi: 10.1111/nin.12313.

Given, C. W., Given, B. A., Stommel, M., & Azzouz, F. (1999). The Impact of New Demands for Assistance on Caregiver Depression: Tests Using an Inception Cohort. *The Gerontologist*, *39*(1), 76–85. doi: 10.1093/geront/39.1.76.

Graafmans, J. A. M. (1992). *Gerontechnology*. Amsterdam: IOS Press.

Gratsa, A., Spiller, M. J., Holt, G., Joyce, T., Hardy, S., & Bouras, N. (2007). Developing a Mental Health Guide for Families and Carers of People with Intellectual Disabilities. *Journal of Applied Research in Intellectual Disabilities*, *20*(2), 77–86. doi: 10.1111/j.1468-3148.2005.00296.x.

Gray, T. F., Nolan, M. T., Clayman, M. L., & Wenzel, J. A. (2019). The decision partner in healthcare decision-making: A concept analysis. *International Journal of Nursing Studies*, *92*, 79–89. doi: 10.1016/j.ijnurstu.2019.01.006.

Hage, A. M., & Lorensen, M. (2005). A philosophical analysis of the concept empowerment; the fundament of an education-programme to the frail elderly. *Nursing Philosophy*, *6*(4), 235–246. doi: 10.1111/j.1466-769x.2005.00231.x.

International Osteoporosis Foundation: *Bone Health*. (n.d.). Retrieved from https://www.iofbonehealth.org/.

Jönsson Ann-Cathrin, Lindgren, I., Hallström Björn, Norrving, B., & Lindgren, A. (2005). Determinants of Quality of Life in Stroke Survivors and Their Informal Caregivers. *Stroke*, *36*(4), 803–808. doi: 10.1161/01.str.0000160873.32791.20.

Kristensen, M. T. (2011). Factors affecting functional prognosis of patients with hip fracture. *European journal of physical and rehabilitation medicine*, 47:257-64, ISSN: 1973-9095.

Larson, J., Franzén-Dahlin, Å., Billing, E., Arbin, M., Murray, V., & Wredling, R. (2005). The impact of a nurse-led support and education programme for spouses of stroke patients: a randomized controlled trial. *Journal of Clinical Nursing*, *14*(8), 995–1003. doi: 10.1111/j.1365-2702.2005.01206.x.

Lin, P.-C., & Lu, C.-M. (2005). Hip fracture: family caregivers' burden and related factors for older people in Taiwan. *Journal of Clinical Nursing*, *14*(6), 719–726. doi: 10.1111/j.1365-2702.2005.01130.x.

Lin, P.-C., & Lu, C.-M. (2007). Psychosocial Factors Affecting Hip Fracture Elder's Burden of Care in Taiwan. *Orthopaedic Nursing*, *26*(3), 155–161. doi: 10.1097/01.nor.0000276964.23270.92.

Liu, H.-Y., Yang, C.-T., Cheng, H.-S., Wu, C.-C., Chen, C.-Y., & Shyu, Y.-I. L. (2015). Family caregivers mental health is associated with postoperative recovery of elderly patients with hip fracture: A sample in Taiwan. *Journal of Psychosomatic Research*, *78*(5), 452–458. doi: 10.1016/j.jpsychores.2015.02.002.

Lloyd, M., & Carson, A. (2005). Culture shift: carer empowerment and cooperative inquiry. *Journal of Psychiatric and Mental Health Nursing*, *12*(2), 187–191. doi: 10.1111/j.1365-2850.2004.00816.x.

Magnusson, L., & Hanson, E. (2005). Supporting frail older people and their family carers at home using information and communication technology: cost analysis. *Journal of Advanced Nursing*, *51*(6), 645–657. doi: 10.1111/j.1365-2648.2005.03541.x.

Mccullagh, E., Brigstocke, G., Donaldson, N., & Kalra, L. (2005). Determinants of Caregiving Burden and Quality of Life in Caregivers of Stroke Patients. *Stroke, 36*(10), 2181–2186. doi: 10.1161/01.str. 0000181755.23914.53.

Mestheneos, E., & Triantafillou, J. (2005). *Supporting Family Carers of Older People in Europe-The Pan-European Backgroung*, pp.160, ISBN: 3-8258-9121-6.

Micera, S., Bonato, P., & Tamura, T. (2008). Gerontechnology. *IEEE Engineering in Medicine and Biology Magazine*, *27*(4), 10–14. doi: 10.1109/memb.2008.925213.

Montgomery, R. J. V., & Kosloski, K. D. (2012). Pathways to a Caregiver Identity and Implications for Support Services. *Caregiving Across the Lifespan Caregiving: Research Practice Policy*, 131–156. doi: 10.1007/978-1-4614-5553-0_8.

Morimoto, T. (2003). Caregiver burden and health-related quality of life among Japanese stroke caregivers. *Age and Ageing*, *32*(2), 218–223. doi: 10.1093/ageing/32.2.218.

Nahm, E.-S., Resnick, B., Orwig, D., Magaziner, J., & Degrezia, M. (2010). Exploration of Informal Caregiving Following Hip Fracture. *Geriatric Nursing*, *31*(4), 254–262. doi: 10.1016/j.gerinurse.2010.01.003.

National Alliance for Caregiving, AARP. Caregiving in the U.S (2004). Bethesda, MD: *National Alliance for Caregiving*. Available from https://www.caregiving.org/.

National Institute for Health and Care Exellence (NICE). (2011). *Hip fracture: management – Clinical Guideline*. Available from www.nice. org.uk/guidance/cg124.

Neugaard, B., Andresen, E., Mckune, S. L., & Jamoom, E. W. (2008). Health-Related Quality of Life in a National Sample of Caregivers: Findings from the Behavioral Risk Factor Surveillance System. *Journal of Happiness Studies*, *9*(4), 559–575. doi: 10.1007/s10902-008-9089-2.

Novak, M., & Guest, C. (1989). Application of a Multidimensional Caregiver Burden Inventory. *The Gerontologist*, *29*(6), 798–803. doi: 10.1093/geront/29.6.798.

Pearlin, L. I., Mullan, J. T., Semple, S. J., & Skaff, M. M. (1990). Caregiving and the Stress Process: An Overview of Concepts and Their Measures. *The Gerontologist*, *30*(5), 583–594. doi: 10.1093/geront/30.5.583.

Raphael, C., & Cornwell, J. L. (2008). Influencing Support for Caregivers. *AJN, American Journal of Nursing*, *108*(Supplement), 78–82. doi: 10.1097/01.naj.0000336428.73064.f4.

Regt, M. D. (2011). Intimate Labors. Cultures, Technologies, and the Politics of Care. Ed. by Eileen Boris and Rhacel Salazar Parreñas. Stanford University Press, Stanford (Cal.) 2010. xiv, 340 pp. *International Review of Social History*, *56*(3), 539–542. doi: 10.1017/s0020859011000599.

Reinhard, S. C., Given, B. & Petlick, N. H. (2008). Supporting Family Caregivers in Providing Care. In: Hughes RG, editor. *Patient Safety and Quality: An Evidence-Based Handbook for Nurses.* Rockville (MD): Agency for Healthcare Research and Quality (US), Chapter 14. Available from: https://www.ncbi.nlm.nih.gov/books/NBK2665/.

Reinhard, S. C. (1994). Living with mental illness: Effects of professional support and personal control on caregiver burden. *Research in Nursing & Health*, *17*(2), 79–88. doi: 10.1002/nur.4770170203.

Rodgers, H., Atkinson, C., Bond, S., Suddes, M., Dobson, R., & Curless, R. (1999). Randomized Controlled Trial of a Comprehensive Stroke Education Program for Patients and Caregivers. *Stroke*, *30*(12), 2585–2591. doi: 10.1161/01.str.30.12.2585.

Roth, D. L., Mittelman, M. S., Clay, O. J., Madan, A., & Haley, W. E. (2005). Changes in social support as mediators of the impact of a psychosocial intervention for spouse caregivers of persons with Alzheimers disease. *Psychology and Aging*, *20*(4), 634–644. doi: 10.1037/0882-7974.20.4.634.

Sakanashi, S., & Fujita, K. (2017). Empowerment of family caregivers of adults and elderly persons: A concept analysis. *International Journal of Nursing Practice*, *23*(5). doi: 10.1111/ijn.12573.

Schulz, R., & Sherwood, P. R. (2008). Physical and Mental Health Effects of Family Caregiving. *AJN, American Journal of Nursing*, *108*(Supplement), 23–27. doi: 10.1097/01.naj.0000336406.45248.4c.

Shyu, Y.-I. L., Chen, M.-C., Liang, J., & Tseng, M.-Y. (2011). Trends in health outcomes for family caregivers of hip-fractured elders during the first 12 months after discharge. *Journal of Advanced Nursing*, *68*(3), 658–666. doi: 10.1111/j.1365-2648.2011.05778.x.

Sinnakaruppan, I., Downey, B., & Morrison, S. (2005). Head injury and family carers: A pilot study to investigate an innovative community-based educational programme for family carers and patients. *Brain Injury*, *19*(4), 283–308. doi: 10.1080/02699050400003924.

Stoltz, P., Uden, G., & Willman, A. (2004). Support for family carers who care for an elderly person at home - A systematic literature review. *Scandinavian Journal of Caring Sciences*, *18*(2), 111–119. doi: 10.1111/j.1471-6712.2004.00269.x.

Teri, L., Mccurry, S. M., Logsdon, R., & Gibbons, L. E. (2005). Training Community Consultants to Help Family Members Improve Dementia Care: A Randomized Controlled Trial. *The Gerontologist*, *45*(6), 802–811. doi: 10.1093/geront/45.6.802.

Thomas, L. C. (2017). Improving Caregiver Knowledge of Support Resources. *Federal practitioner: For the health care professionals of the VA, DoD, and PHS*, *34*(3), 45–48.

Torp, S., Hanson, E., Hauge, S., Ulstein, I., & Magnusson, L. (2007). A pilot study of how information and communication technology may contribute to health promotion among elderly spousal carers in Norway. *Health & Social Care in the Community*, *16*(1), 75–85. doi: 10.1111/j.1365-2524.2007.00725.x.

Wallsten, S. S. (2000). Effects of Caregiving, Gender, and Race on the Health, Mutuality, and Social Supports of Older Couples. *Journal of Aging and Health*, *12*(1), 90–111. doi: 10.1177/089826430001200105.

Yeates, N. (2012). Global care chains: a state-of-the-art review and future directions in care transnationalization research. *Global Networks*, *12*(2), 135–154. doi: 10.1111/j.1471-0374.2012.00344.x.

Young, Y., Xiong, K., & Pruzek, R. M. (2011). Longitudinal Functional Recovery after Postacute Rehabilitation in Older Hip Fracture Patients: The Role of Cognitive Impairment and Implications for Long-Term

Care. *Journal of the American Medical Directors Association, 12*(6), 431–438. doi: 10.1016/j.jamda.2010.08.005.

Zarit, S. H., Stephens, M. A. P., Townsend, A., & Greene, R. (1998). Stress Reduction for Family Caregivers: Effects of Adult Day Care Use. *The Journals of Gerontology. Series B: Psychological Sciences and Social Sciences, 53B*(5). doi: 10.1093/geronb/53b.5.s267.

In: Caregiving
Editor: Stefano Eleuteri

ISBN: 978-1-53616-889-1

Chapter 5

IN CAREGIVERS' HANDS: INTERPERSONAL TOUCH AND CONTACT WITHIN CARING

Enrico De Luca*

Department of Developmental and Social Psychology,
University 'La Sapienza' Rome, Italy

ABSTRACT

Since the '60s several studies have been showing the importance of touch, especially within the caring relationship and healthcare settings. Touch is the sense of reciprocity, a fundamental axiom affirms that: "we can't touch without being touched". Moreover, the interest in formal or informal caregivers' well-being and psychosocial functioning has already highlighted the fragility of this caring position. Since Touching is unavoidable in Caring, formal and informal caregivers might benefit from an implemented awareness of the impact of their touch style and the way they intend physical contact. In addition, caregivers' education has a pivotal role in reducing their burn-out and compassion fatigue. Thus, it can

* Corresponding Author's Email: enrico.deluca@uniroma1.it.

be hypothesized a model of intervention (on social scale or family-oriented) to support who cares for others that are living in a situation of frailty (such as: older citizens, persons with disability, end of life care and/or children) and help them to build together a corporeal vocabulary where the word "Caring" regains its original meaning.

Keywords: interpersonal touch, caring relationship, physical contact, massage, healthcare touch studies

INTRODUCTION

This contribution first started as a reflection on the weight of the noun *Care* in the term Care-giving. In fact, the noun Care (and from this the verb to Care) originally has several meanings and an interesting etymology, and this can help us to understand the fundamentals of this art. Moreover, the act of exploring the meanings of Care itself could also be a way to suggest an improvement and to look at Caregiving from a different perspective. In addition to this, it must be considered that, just as the Latin myth of Care (Cura) suggests that to "take care of" is about creating Life with the hands and gestures, Caregiving implies mostly to touch patients. Caregiving for long-term, disabled and dependent elderly citizens means direct care mostly mediated by touch; especially in these contexts and settings, touch can be used as an important patient comforting tool as well as for physical and hygiene care. Touch is unavoidable and it is the sense of the reciprocity but how many caregivers (and healthcare professionals) are aware of influence and power of their touch? For this reason, the importance of interpersonal touch in healthcare will be highlighted and discussed. In addition to this, recent findings have shown that healthcare professionals' touch style can influence their caring attitude and also their tendency to have work-related stress. From here it can be hypothesized that caregivers could benefit from a better attitude towards touch and an understanding of the fundamentals of care, to lessen their physical and emotional burden. This leads us to argue that caregivers' education, lifelong learning, specific training and support can be crucial for their psycho-physical wellbeing and patients' healthcare.

However, caregiving scenarios in Italy depict a large number of "hidden workers" and, something that is difficult to trace, direct care provided in the private sector. A last reflection can be made on the fact that maybe it is still possible to educate to care, and what's more, that we can help those who "care for the others" to learn how to touch in a caring and humane manner.

THE PRIMACY OF CARING

"Caring is not optional, it is something that is natural and obligatory (for which loving is another word) is to be involved, intimate".

(Montagu, 1971, p. 282).

Caring permeates every aspect of our life but, in a healthcare setting, we can witness the creation of a specific 'relational space', often non-verbal and with its own proxemic, that has been at the center of the reflections and thoughts of psychologists, philosophers, social scientist and researchers.

To have an understanding of what Caring means and to define it, we need to look back to the roots of the term Care. It must be said that Caring theories have been at the center of Nursing studies, therefore I will use them as a resource for reflections on Caregiving, especially formal and professional. The primacy of Care, and hence of caring (Benner, Tanner and Chelsea, 2009), constitutes a basic axiom upon which considerations have arisen and nurse scientists (like nursing theorists: Jean Watson[1], Sally Gadow[2] and Madeleine Leininger[3]) have built the foundations for a meaningful theoretical framework (Blasdell, 2017).

The word "care" is itself a term of polysemantic characteristics, with different meanings and possibilities of interpretation. Among its several

---

[1] Dr. Jean Watson explored and created the Human Caring Theory in Nursing. https://www.watsoncaringscience.org/

[2] Professor Emerita Sally Gadow (Colorado University-USA) has contributed with profound insights on concepts of advocacy and caring in nursing theories.

[3] Professor Emerita Madeleine Leininger (1925 –2012) developed the concept of transcultural nursing theory and explored the meaning of caring.

meanings, we can find: thought for someone, interest, concern, commitment for someone or something, anxiety or fear for, raising and cultivating[4].

The Italian word for care is *Cura* and, once entering the medical field, it represents a real and proper therapeutic action and a special attention to those who are experiencing moments of fragility too (Reich, 1995; Grassi, 2013). Thus, in Italian, we find enclosed in one word the two existing tensions described by the meaning of care, which is anxiety on one side and affection on the other. An important distinction, that can contribute to better understand the weight of Care in Caregiving, comes from the English language and it is the difference between the use of two verbs: *to cure* and *to care.*

In fact, Nursing studies and Medical philosophy have been concerned with long debates and radical questions about the sense of caring and curing, a sense that has been historically overlapped or counterposed (Jecker & Self, 1991). From this perspective, to cure or curing concerns the activity of treating the diseases of the body, an act that is above all medical and linked to therapeutic practices, whereas to care or caring represents a cure that deals with the other, which is not just a "repair" of something that does not work, but the care of being in its complexity (Kleinman & Van Der Geest, 2009; Mortari & Saiani 2014).

Italian epistemologist Luigina Mortari (2014) states that we can find the concept of care in the work *Being in time* (2011) of the philosopher Martin Heidegger (1889-1976). Heidegger affirms that *being-in-the-world* is essentially caring; the German philosopher uses mythology[5] as a metaphor to describe clearly that Care (or *Cura*, from the Latin Myth) exists before

---

[4] https://dictionary.cambridge.org/dictionary/english/care.

[5] As Care (Cura) was crossing a river, she thoughtfully picked up some mud and began to fashion a human being. While she was pondering what she had done, Jupiter came along. Care asked him to give the spirit of life to the human being, and Jupiter readily granted this. Care wanted to name the human after herself, but Jupiter insisted that his name should be given to the human instead. While Care and Jupiter were arguing, Terra arose and said that the human being should be named after her, since she had given her own body. Finally, all three disputants accepted Saturn as a judge. Saturn decided that Jupiter, who gave spirit to the human, would take back its soul after death; and since Terra had offered her body to the human, she should receive it back after death. But, said Saturn, "Since Care first fashioned the human being, let her have and hold it as long as it lives". Finally, Jupiter said, "Let it be called homo (Latin for human being), since it seems to be made from humus (Latin for earth)" (Heidegger, 2011, pp 282-283).

Being, that Care precedes Being. So, Care shapes (the) Being. Receiving care is the necessary condition to open up the 'possibilities of being'. Thus, without the nourishment of Care life ceases to exist. In this sense, Heidegger speaks of the *ontological primacy of care.* Care is a fundamental way of being, because, to realize human life, we all need both to be the object of care and to care for others.

Caring as a Practice

Heidegger (2011) affirms that to take care (expressed as the welfare work) is based on a constitution of a being (called Dasein[6]) intended as "being-with"; thus, our "being in the world" takes place through establishing relationships with others. Therefore, humankind has the absolute need to receive care and, at the same time, needs to take care of itself, of others and the world, in order to understand the meaning of its existence. In fact, Mortari (2013) highlights that theories that intend to support the thesis of the primacy of caring also need to consider care as a practice directed to others (and therefore to a relationship). The other that *pre-exists* us, that precedes us and that has taken care of us, to allow us to continue to be there. Mortari (2013) cites French philosopher Levinàs (1904-1996) and introduces the concept of "caring for others" as a practice that qualifies a profession; as it is necessary, for the practice of care itself, to feel an obligation towards the other, since "we never exist in the singular". A relationship in which the other is left free to be totally different from us.

From here, the "sense of the other" will always be present, even in our corporeality, in our bodily perception; it is always the other, in a certain way, that shapes our being, through its caresses, love and even, unfortunately, the beatings and injuries (Marzano, 2007). These premises inevitably draw back into a "primary dimension" where we have been the object of cares; a special dimension where our personal and unique relationship with those who took

[6] In Being and Time, Heidegger (2011, 29-30) "…the ontological character of Dasein (…) does not signify being but rather being in the manner of an understanding being". The term Dasein has been chosen by the philosopher to designate an existential experience of being.

care of us, especially from birth and the first moments of our lives, represents a model and offers an important imprint for future caregiving relationships.

The concept of care can thus be summarized in three possible natures. The first has a cognitive nature: caring for someone means thinking about him/her, keeping the other in mind. The second of passionate nature: caring for someone means feeling an interest, paying attention, feeling anxiety. The third is between cognition and passion and it is action. This last happens when Care is realized in terms of a practice or an act where conceived thoughts, intentionality, emotions are directed towards the object of care, helping the other to become him/herself or to develop his/her possible being (Mortari & Saiani, 2014; Heidegger, 2011).

Gestures of Care

> *"If we accept that Care is an ontological necessity and that caring for, which authenticates human life, must be learned, then care must have an important place in the education field"*
>
> (Mortari, 2004, pp. 109-122).

All care interventions can morph into care gestures, but this requires a change of perspective. Such a shift can materialize once we assume a different posture, not only physical but also intellectual, within a caring relationship. This implies adopting a mental posture that fosters our abilities to listen, to self-investigate and then to move towards, so as to come intentionally in contact with the other. From a philosophical stand point, in intentionality, there is a mental movement that goes from the concept and representation towards the object[7].

In other words, that necessary *Being-with*, in the relationship with the world, which has the capacity to change the very "substance of the encounter" (Heidegger, 2011). The philosophical current of phenomenology describes intentionality as a thought's constitutive attitude to always having

---

[7] https://plato.stanford.edu/entries/intentionality/

a content and of necessarily going towards an object; hence a thought without intentionality would not exist (Merleau-Ponty, 2013).

Several researchers have emphasized that, when there is intentionality in caring practice, one comes into contact with the other, recognizing and meeting not only a body but a person (Chang, 2001; Connor & Howett, 2009). Fredriksson (1999), in his study on caring, presence and intentionality, draws attention to the fact that the carer is often in a position that allows him/her to transform a "being there" into a "being with", creating connection and intersubjectivity.

Therefore, the human action has the possibility of becoming an intentional action, that intentionality which the human being perceives as original and primary. Mortari (2014) quotes the Aristotelian principle that "everything tends to good", and thus every being is moved by the intention to seek the good. Aristotle (384–322 BC) specifies that this good is called eudaimonia which literally means to live in a good dimension of the spirit (Huta, 2013). Therefore, the intention that sustains a good care practice will deal with what makes us live well, having clear the premises of the ontological primacy of care and an eudaimonistic intentionality of being (Nussbaum, 2001).

Based on these assumptions, the gesture of care can be defined as an "*intentional gesture that aims at the well-being of the individual*".

Caring and Touch

Touching and contact are fundamental features of caregiving. It has been estimated that 85% of caring for an elderly patient involves touching (Grousset, 2009). Providing physical comfort, personal hygiene, changing position in bed or helping to mobilize from bed to chair and vice-versa, and support for ambulation are the most usual tasks for caregiving in this setting.

Other implicit touching situations are not taken into account, such as: helping to get dressed, to use rehabilitative support, to eat, to read. These actions are often referred to as implicit care (Canzan, Heilemann, Saiani, Mortari, & Ambrosi 2014). Hence, to explore the meaning of touch, from a different point of view, can give an insight into the importance of interpersonal touch and contact within caregiving.

Touch: A Multidimensional Sense

Our sense of touch leads us into a realm of complex reflections; such reflections have inspired scientific theories and psychoanalytic schools and have guided discoveries in the fields of social and cognitive psychology, neuroscience and cultural anthropology. Describing the sense of touch means, first of all, to focus on our body and corporeality; in fact, touch is in some way 'constitutive' of bodily experience in ways that other senses are not (Lindgren, Westling, Brulin, Lehtipalo, Andersson & Nyberg, 2012; Serino & Haggard, 2010; de Vignemont, 2010). Being part of the physical world involves coming into physical contact with things and objects and therefore touch is the most important sense, the essential sense for having a body, for being able to interact with what we are surrounded by (Fulkerson, 2014). The peculiar functional duplicity of tactile perception that incorporates, in a single sensory system, the apprehension of external things and the interoceptive functions, gives rise to the experience of the body felt "from within" (Fugali, 2012). Wehrle (2018) quoting Edmund Husserl (1859-1938) affirms that from a cognitive point of view, the capacity of being able to be touched and to touch gives to the body the possibility of being simultaneously an object and an *openness* to the world itself, so to speak, a lived body and living body. In addition to this, Maurice Merleau-Ponty (1908-1961) with a phenomenological approach, projects the body into a world of relationships and sensations, where the "body that feels" and the "body sensed" represent two sides of the same coin (Marzano, 2007).

During the twentieth century, currents of thoughts and schools of psychoanalysis and psychotherapy have been interested in developing models where the body, and hence the skin and contact, represents a way to access, understand and express the psychic world. The studies of the major theorists on attachment and child development have constantly highlighted the fundamental importance of interpersonal contact; among the most important scientists and psychoanalysts interested in touch, we have John Bowlby, Mary Ainsworth, Donald Winnicott, Harry Harlow, René Spitz, and Didier Anzieu.

We owe to the anthropologist Ashley Montagu (1905-1999) a study on the language of the skin that has influenced a whole generation of research up to our days. Montagu, in *Touching: the human significance of the skin* (1971), focuses his study on how the tactile experience, or a lack of it, affects the development of behavior, of the person and their fundamental psychophysiological processes, also extending to cultural and social implications. He demonstrates, through an analysis of numerous researches, that there is an indelible "memory of the skin" in each of us, which starts from our intrauterine life. The contact, the caresses, the massage already in the first moments of life have measurable effects on physiological well-being, ranging from the weight gain of premature babies to the improvement of the immune system and a more harmonious general development.

Montagu (1971) defines the memory of the skin as a real language: "If it is true that this language is structured as children, it is the experiences of all life that enrich or impoverish it. The need for caresses, if it is vital for the child, remains indispensable for life (some elderly people let themselves die if abruptly deprived of contact and recognition to which they are accustomed)" (p. 100). Therefore, contact is probably the best form of communication that is present and possible, available to us, in the care of the infant and of the dying person. The psychiatrist Kübler-Ross (1926-2004), in her fundamental study on death and dying, described in great detail how, being present with the touch, of a gentle and firm hand, is the best way to communicate at the end of life (Kübler-Ross & Kessler, 2005).

In the last three decades, the studies of social and cognitive psychology have been interested in interpersonal contact and communication in adults; through empirical research and social experiments the importance of this sense has been unveiled. Hertenstein et al. (2006), exploring the literature and research on contact, underlined how numerous behaviors, such as modulating the tendency to fulfill a task, the attitude towards specific services, creating bonds between couples and groups or simply strengthening romantic relationships, are influenced by a contact experience.

It should be added that this influence occurs whether the experience of interpersonal contact is explicitly remembered or not by the individuals involved (Hertenstein, Verkamp, Kerestes & Holmes, 2006). They cited a research by Fisher, Rytting & Heslin (1976) which is one the most classical and influential on this subject. This study has shown how the (unaware) touch of the staff of a library of an American university faculty was a determining factor in the satisfaction of the student, who had benefited from that service (Fisher, Rytting & Heslin, 1976). Gallace and Spence (2010) collected decisive evidence of touch's persuasive potential, also when it is unaware interpersonal contact. In fact, they illustrate several touch researches conducted by social-scientists focused on customer compliance services or commercial activities, and also on the scholastic participation of students or the enjoyment of a service. The increased level of compliance, generosity or good predisposition towards the other implies that a social and rudimental touch could also constitute a basis for trust and cooperation, in possible future exchanges (Morrison, Löken & Olausson, 2010). According to Hertnstein et al. (2006) contact offers opportunities to communicate emotions and thoughts; for this group of scholars, tactile communication is understood as "a systematic change in the individual of his perceptions, thoughts, feelings or behavior according to the touch of another and in relation to the context in which this occurs" (p. 8). Hertenstein, Keltner, App, Bulleit & Jaskolka (2006) have shown, with the hypothesis of a contact aimed at the emotional aspect, how individuals (of two different nationalities) can discriminate different emotions and feelings on the basis of how they were touched. In this study, two different groups were blindfolded and touched on the forearm; the touches were of different styles (from a sharp touch to a caress) and participants' descriptions of their emotions and feelings aroused by each type of touch were recorded, using a predominantly quantitative approach.

The hypotheses on contact and the emotional world have also been revisited by social scientists and neuroscientists in more recent periods, supporting the idea that the typology of touch is influenced by the different neuronal possibilities or the transmission and processing of the nerve itself (Gallace & Spence, 2010). The advent of new neuroimaging techniques has made this kind of research possible and also the different insights into physical contact and nerve fibers appointed to different types of tactile sensations. In this current of studies, the existence and correlations of specialized nerve fibers and specific neuronal pathways (from different cutaneous receptors to upper nerve centers to intermediate and cortical brain areas) have been traced based on the different modes of touch. Further and consistent evidence, which emerges from numerous biographical testimonies, transposed into literature and even into cinematography, highlights the experience of patients in a state (of different types) of coma and their bodily memories. The body and the skin have a memory of what is happening, our body "remembers" even when the highest cortical level of consciousness seems to have ceased to function; at the somatosensory level, physical and psychological traumas remain as a real imprint in the body (Ogden, Minton & Pain, 2006). Cognitive neuroscience has found that in the quality of contact, in addition to the pleasure and the hedonistic aspect of the experience, the stimulus directed to the brain area of affectivity, once it is contacted and consequently elicits responses, is a discriminating factor. In fact, there are specific pathways for affectivity and touch; in other words, the brain is able to distinguish the affective aspects of a touch from emotionally neutral tactile sensations (McGlone, Vallbo, Olausson, Loken & Wessberg, 2007; Olausson, Cole, Rylander, McGlone, Lamarre, Wallin & Vallbo, 2008). These 'affective' fibers, so named by neuroscientists, carry information directly into areas of the brain close to the limbic system, and they elaborate the stimulus for an innate process, thus not for a previously interpreted or learned process. This is like the stimuli mediated by other afferent and faster "touch fibers", which instead reach the somatosensory cortex, and are therefore linked to analytical processes that depend on previous tactile experiences (Lindgren et al., 2012; Croy, Sehlstedt, Wasling, Ackerley, & Olausson, 2017). It has been highlighted that these affective fibers (or C-fibers) convey specific information related to emotions, compared to other fibers that have the ability to transport sensations of a physical state (McGlone, Wessberg & Olausson 2014).

All this goes even further to support those researches in the field of cognitive and social neuroscience that support the assumption that interpersonal tactile stimulation is an effective means to influence the social and affective behavior of individuals as well as contributing to body memory (Gallace & Spence, 2010).

Interpersonal Touch in Healthcare

The topic of touch and its fundamental importance in the relational and communicative aspects within the healthcare context, seems to have occupied little space among the research fields of classical medicine (Hertenstein et al., 2006). By contrast, researches and studies conducted by direct care professionals seem to be more interested in the topic of touch. Montagu (1971) states that "... *a branch of the health community that has recognized the importance of touch is the nursing profession. Many articles on the effects of contact have already appeared in nursing publications. Being so close to the patient as compared to the doctor has put the nurse in the preferential position to appreciate the importance of contact into patient care and that treatment begins with caring*" (p. 282).

A previous exploratory literature review, conducted in a doctoral program, confirmed that, compared to scientific medical research tout court, nursing research has always been interested in interpersonal contact. In fact, there are very few medical researches devoted exclusively to aspects related to contact or interpersonal contact.

More specifically, observing the categories that emerged and comparing the results of the research, it has been possible to elicit the following observations:

1. the areas where studies have been done are mostly intensive care, pediatrics, geriatrics, hospice care and palliative care (McCann & McKenna, 1993; Routasalo & Isola, 1998; Grousset, 2009; Gleeson & Timmins, 2004);
2. reference is made to contact with the patient in the medical literature of family doctors as a topic of interest for family medicine or in

some manuals for family medical students (Cocksedge, George, Renwick & Chew-Graham, 2013);
3. broad interest in interpersonal contact in psychology, psychoanalysis or psychiatry journals (Salzmann-Erikson & Eriksson, 2005);
4. other health professionals such as rehabilitation therapists, obstetricians, occupational therapists and caregivers are scarcely present (Hertenstein et al., 2006).

It has been noticed that, according to diverse methodologies and approaches used in empirical research, there has been a semantic evolution of definitions and terms concerning contact in the context of care. The first researches from the 60s to the 80s were interested in quantitative aspects of the phenomenon of contact, focusing on measuring the features and use of touch in healthcare settings. Routasalo (1999) states that contact research, in nursing sciences, had an initial moment (from the 1960s) where a quantitative approach was important since it was more concerned with how many times and where the contact took place. In fact, the research on contact has focused primarily on categorizing all types of touch or contact that the nurse acts in the context, such as completing a task or giving comfort to the patient (Weiss & Niemann, 2011). Contact as a measure of the nurse's presence in the care relationship is the subject of the study by Fredriksson (1999). According to Fredriksson (1999), from an ontological point of view, contact, presence and listening are phenomena that connect individuals. A mutual connection that allows different degrees of intersubjectivity. In his contact summary, he analyzes 11 qualitative studies and synthesizes 108 excerpts from studies, thus building a structure where touch in the care relationship is defined as 'contact' and/or 'contact without touch'. In Fredriksson, the contact is subdivided according to the model proposed by Estabrooks and Morse (1992) that is: a task-oriented contact, a contact as a form of non-verbal communication of feelings and sensations (caring and connection) and a contact as a strategy to protect the nurse from an emotional overload or suffering (protective). In Fredriksson's reflections, it is highlighted how the caring relationship is characterized by a 'high intensity' intersubjectivity as opposed to simple contact as a relationship of reduced intensity and with fewer characteristics of intersubjectivity.

Chang (2001), in a study aimed at designing a conceptual structure of contact in healthcare, determines five types of contacts defined as a touch "in caring situations", eventually coming to show contact essentially as intentional or unintentional. Indeed, the scholar, observing how complex it is to study a phenomenon where the elements of subjectivity are strong, built a conceptual model on the physical contact in caring, both thinking of it as a phenomenon and as different possibilities or methods of treatment. In Chang's model (2001), contact takes place in five different ways, each of which in turn belongs to a human dimension: physical, emotional, social and spiritual. Some of the five modes can cross different dimensions and overlap giving a final picture of the contact in caring as a human phenomenon that can integrate the different types (for example in the task-orientated touch mode there can be not only the physical dimension but also the emotional dimension). Contact studies have spread in the geriatric context, aimed at demonstrating the effects of this on the elderly person considered to be often deprived both emotionally and sensorially (Gleeson & Timmins, 2004; Grousset, 2009). In this regard, Montagu (1971) often speaks of the deprivation of skin contact of the elderly, as their skin is no longer touched or even considered touchable. The studies of Gleeson & Timmins (2004, 2005) are addressed to a particular group of patients with dementia and are designed to show how the use of an "expressive touch" (term first introduced by McCann & McKenna in 1993) can improve their emotional well-being. The elderly patient with dementia is a patient who often loses the ability to communicate effectively; therefore, contact will remain a vital constant for these patients. The expressive touch, illustrated by Gleeson & Timmins (2004, 2005), could be used to infuse emotions and caring, establish contact with the patient, reassure and comfort in stressful situations. Grousset (2009) in measuring the opportunities for contact between nurse and patient, specifically in geriatric care, notes that about 85% of nursing practice includes touch or/and entering into contact with the patient. A touch or contact that also occurs unknowingly and/or unintentionally. Leonard and Kalman (2015) observe, as for Chang (2001), that what allows us to cross the limits of the task-oriented touch to go towards a caring contact is actually the relationship. In fact, they adopt different definitions of touch, also quoting Gadow's definition of an 'empathic' touch as a contact acted in the context of "intersubjectivity, a touch that affirms in the patient the dignity and sense of value that morally distinguishes people from objects" (Gadow, 1984, p.512). Kelly, Nixon, McClurg, Scherpbier, King, & Dornan (2018) carried out a meta-ethnographic review of the literature, with research on the themes of contact in the health professions. In the review, they offer a vision of contact in care contexts as a multi-faceted phenomenon and underline how contact is a space where it is possible to communicate "beyond words" (Kelly et al., 2018 p. 206).

From this brief and not yet exhaustive overview of touch, an attempt can be made to summarize all the definitions encountered. Thus, contact in the context of healthcare, besides being a fundamental element for non-verbal communication, can have the following characteristics: intentional or unintentional; procedural, instrumental or task-oriented; empathic, affective, expressive, for emotional containment, compassionate; protective.

A reflection on this review highlights the absence of studies concerned with a specific contact education or training for the healthcare professional, and what's more, very few studies focused on caregiving and touch. Although there are several documented experiences related to contact education via complementary care (Field, 2016) there seem to be very few conceptual or operational models of care where the practice of an intentional, aware contact, or a reflective model on how to get in touch with the other, are taken into account. Finally, it is interesting to note that in the Italian panorama, some studies and nursing scientific research on contact have been emerging just in the last decade.

Touch and Work-Related Stress

Most of the literature on contact examined up to now is focused on describing the quality of this touch, the effect on patients or the carer-patient relationship. Among the very few studies concerned with interpersonal touch, healthcare professional well-being and work-related stress prevention, two recent researches can be mentioned for their effort in this direction. An Italian research (Pedrazza, Berlanda, Trifiletti &Minuzzo, 2015; 2018) hypothesized a correlation between comfort with interpersonal touch and work well-being. The study by Pedrazza et al. (2015) on nurses' organizational well-being and comfort with touch followed 241 nurses participating in a company refresher course on pain management. In this quantitative study, the tools used are Comfort with Touch' Scale, Maslach Burnout Inventory and a Job Satisfaction scale. The results indicated that there was a positive correlation between comfort with touch and work well-being while suggesting that contact discomfort is related to burnout and low job satisfaction. Specifically, there are high probabilities (according to this hypothesized model) of a strong relationship between contact difficulties to provide emotional support and cynicism, which is thought to be a predictive factor for burn-out (Pedrazza et al., 2015). A recent study focusing on US nurses who have undergone training in massage techniques, observed the training effect on burn-out, compassion fatigue, and work well-being (Wilson, Gettel, Walsh & Esquenazi, 2016). In a southwestern U.S. acute care hospital system, 30 nurses undertook the training and massaged their patients over a period of 8 weeks. Nurses completed two questionnaires, respectively: ProQool - a validated tool to measure compassion satisfaction, burnout and perceived stress; the Nyberg Caring Assessment Scala (CAS), a scale for measuring perceived caring. The study gave results in terms of better job satisfaction and a reduction in compassion fatigue among nurses who massaged. On the other hand, a significant positive relationship was found between the Caring scale and compassion satisfaction, whereas a negative correlation was found between Caring and Burnout values. Furthermore, nurses who participated in the project reported a greater sense of the profession: the massage allowed them to approach the patient differently.

CAREGIVERS' JOB

According to the standard definition (from European[8] and American Associations'[9] specialised websites and official reports) a caregiver generally is the person providing help to someone with a chronic illness, disability or other long-lasting health or care needs. International literature states an important distinction between formal (therefore professional, paid and/or supported by national or private healthcare systems) and informal (generally unpaid help and/or family members) caregiving. In Italy the term *caregiver* has been introduced recently and most of the time is meant to describe a family member rather than a health professional or paid helper, whereas in Italian a word commonly used for paid, private or generic caregiving (often without qualification) is carer or "badante" (Paniccia, Giovagnoli & Caputo, 2015).).

Caregiving for elderly citizens has been a fast-growing 'caring profile' in industrialized countries; multiple factors have contributed to this phenomenon such as prolonged life expectancy, reduced mortality, better disease prevention and an increase of chronic disease (Moroni, Sguazzin, Filipponi, Bruletti, Callegari, Galante, Majani & Bertolotti, 2008; Rodriguez & Barbagallo, 2012). Besides, the caring demand for a rapidly aging population is a challenge for both formal and informal caregiving. Population aging has a deep influence on family (and other members of a patient's social network) availability for caring, and therefore the reduced ratio between potential informal caregivers to older persons will probably bring a scarcity of informal care (Gaugler, Pestka, Davila, Sales, Owen, Baumgartner, Shook, Cunningham & Kenney, 2018).

Having said that, the prevision of a worldwide massive population ageing brings issues on how formal care will face the scarce informal caregivers, and so how the experience and needs of elderly citizens will influence society (Genet, Boerma, Kroneman, Hutchinson & Saltman, 2012). The increasing number of individuals with chronic functional or

[8] http://ec.europa.eu/social/BlobServlet?docId=12633&langId=en; https://eurocarers.org/

[9] https://www.caregiving.org/research/caregivingusa/

cognitive impairments will influence the rise of the demand for Long Term Care (LTC) (Bruni & Ugolini, 2016). Suanet, van Groenou & Van Tilburg (2012) have observed the different formal and informal care between six European countries; in their study, they have shown problematic issues related to "care workers' "availability, qualifications, and working conditions. From north to south Europe, the care sector has changed in the last decades, creating new forms of employment. In Italy, Austria, and Germany a private care sector, not controlled by social and labor regulations, has emerged. In fact, usually, the family resort to care workers who were once relatively cheap, and undocumented immigrant labor is available (Suanet et al., 2012). Also, social and political support to informal caregiving varies from country to country, but the creation of specific schemes to help families has been part of most European countries' welfare and national health programs (Da Roit & Le Bihan, 2010; Genet et al., 2012).

Formal and informal caregiving (as for all health, psychological, social support and medical professions) means to face personal health and social issues too; in fact, a high level of caring stress is associated with high risk of burn out and poor health (Barbabella, Poli, Andréasson, Salzmann, Papa, Hanson, Lancioni, Eftimiou, Dohner, Civerchia & Lamura, 2016; Cianfrocca, Caponnetto, Donati, Lancia, Tartaglini & Di Stasio, 2018; Fianco, Sartori, Negri, Lorini, Valle & Delle Fave, 2015). The prevalence of mental health problems among caregivers seems to be higher than among non-caregivers, especially in terms of the use of medications, anxiety and depression (Eleuteri, Norton, Livi, Grano, Lucidi, Violani & Lombardo, 2018; Fianco et al., 2015). The well-known "caregiver burden" is the result of the constant involvement in practical and emotional tasks and the perception that caregiving negatively affects the caregiver's life (Adelman, Tmanova, Delgado, Dion & Lachs, 2014; Cianfrocca et al., 2018; Tan, Molassiotis, Lloyd-Williams & Yorke, 2017). Caregiving is also particularly challenging due to difficulties in reconciling care with family activities and social life (Fianco et al., 2015). Gaugler et al. (2018) highlight that the burden for familial caregivers comes also from the difficulties of balancing caregiving and work responsibilities and a lack of flexibility. According to the report "Caregiving in the U.S. 2015", (by the National Alliance for

Caregiving and American Association of Retired Persons)[10] informal caregiving and family members are the most present form of caregiving in the Country. Besides, most of the caregivers (predominantly women) balance work with looking after their relatives; therefore, considering overall caregiver health and well-being, caregiving–work conflict appears to be more relevant to caregiver burden in the US (Gaugler et al., 2018).

Caregivers in Italy

In Italy, throughout the last two decades, caregiving has been a growing phenomenon also for the well-known social and cultural changes in family structure and availability of new immigrants more willing to embrace caregiving as a profession (Nobili, Massaia, Isaia, Cappa, Pilon, Mondino, Bo & Isaia, 2011). Although the Italian family represented for a long time the "caring agency", where unpaid informal care by family members was largely present (Da Roit & Le Bihan, 2010) nowadays, especially elderly care, is increasingly delegated to privately paid caregivers.

According to ISTAT[11], the Italian LCT system has a big contribution from the informal caregivers; in fact, there are about 3.3 million family caregivers, 8.6% of the adult Italian population. Having said that, the family faces increasing difficulties in ensuring the levels of assistance the elderly population requires. Ongoing socio-demographic changes like fewer family ties, the increased presence of women in the labor force, and the availability of formal care alternatives are challenges for informal caregiving, and thus LTC is increasingly delegated to privately paid caregivers (Bruni & Ugolini, 2016). This personal services market, largely based on an unskilled female immigrant workforce, has ensured to many Italian families a substitute for professional home care services, and thus it has had an effect in attenuating the demand for admissions to assisted living facilities (Paniccia et al., 2014). On the other hand, several reports have shown that Italian formal elderly and

[10]https://www.aarp.org/content/dam/aarp/ppi/2015/caregiving-in-the-united-states-2015-report-revised.pdf.

[11] Istat: Italian Institute for Statistics. https://www.istat.it/en/.

LTC care, provided by institutions or at home, is often marginal, it changes from north to south, and services are administered mainly at the regional, local level, with few resources available (Bruni & Ugolini, 2016; Paniccia et al., 2014). Barbabella et al. (2013) and Di Rosa, Barbabella, Chiatti, Melchiorre & Lamura (2013) state that Italy, as one of the oldest and fastest aging Countries in the world, is characterized by one of the highest and fastest increasing demands for elderly care in the world but, paradoxically, also by a surprisingly low level of public provision in this sector. Indeed, the role of formal care services in Italy remains underdeveloped and unequally distributed throughout the Country.

A recent Italian government reform, in order to align with EU regulations, has provided an economic plan to support family caregivers; an act that means an official recognition of psycho-social and financial costs sustained by caregivers[12]. At the same time, several national and regional government reforms have been made, in order to find a way to regulate the carers work market and to reduce undeclared labor, such as: fiscal incentives to facilitate the issuing of contracts, the granting of regular residence permits and immigration quotas to "care" migrants, introducing training and accreditation programs (Di Rosa et al., 2013; Paniccia et al., 2014;).

This briefly outlined overview on informal and formal caregiving has served to introduce the topic of the impact of caregivers' education and from here the education and awareness on touch.

Supporting Caregiver Education

Understanding caregiver learning needs is crucial, especially to plan any educational intervention or possible and achievable trajectories for a training program. Many caregivers, in fact, assume the caregiver role with little or no preparation and have to learn to deal with the many aspects of care in a very short time (Eleuteri, Bellanti & Falaschi, 2016). A recent systematic

---

[12] The Italian Budget Law of 2018 established, in paragraph 254, at the Ministry of Labor and Social Policies the "Fund for the role of care and assistance of the family caregiver. From G.U. Serie generale n. 302 del 29-12-17 – Suppl. Ord. n. 62.

review on the burden of the caregiver suggested several interventions to support caregivers, in order to cope with problems of stress and health. The most important are: encouraging health professionals to become active members of the care team; improving self-care and maintaining one's health; providing education and information; the use of technology support; coordinating/consulting care with care and encouraging healthcare professionals to access respite care (Adelman et al., 2014). Aksoydan, Aytar, Blazeviciene, van Bruchem-Visser, Vaskelyte, Mattace-Raso, Acar, Altinas, Akgun-Citak, Attene-Ozden, Kiziltan & Baskici (2019) confirm the paramount role of training and education, especially in terms of how informal caregivers could have a better quality of life if they have access to supportive educative learning. On the other hand, informal caregiving, apart from direct care, implies the task to support the continuity of care and to have good communication with the formal/professional care team. If caregivers are properly informed, they become more confident in their abilities and they improve their coping skills in managing disease-related problems (Cianfrocca et al., 2018). Therefore, caregiver training might have advantages of reducing health care costs, caregiver anxiety and stress and could help to create better social relations with the care receiver (Williams, 2018; Aksoydan et al., 2019).

Having said that, the inclusion of caregiver "health literacy" as the pivotal role to improve the health of both cared ones and caregiver should be a priority for public health policy (Yuen, Knight, Ricciardelli & Burney, 2018). The Italian government and especially regional districts' healthcare institutions are increasingly investing in caregiver education and support to improve citizens' homecare for all types of disabilities. Initiatives have been introduced to support caregiver education (directed to family members but also carers) with courses offered by the local/district healthcare service. In Rome (like the experience for Tuscany or Emilia Romagna district) there is an ongoing healthcare campaign to offer free courses for caregivers' education. Courses led by volunteer healthcare professionals (from medical, nursing, psychologist and social assistance profiles) who teach caregivers how to deal with home care and other everyday issues[13]. The Nursing Department of "Campus Bio-Medico" of Rome has promoted training courses for family caregivers since 2011 with the intention of supporting families in the acquisition of specific skills related to health care of patients with chronic conditions (Pennacchini, Petriccione, Sisto, Di Santo & Tartaglini, 2014).

These examples of training highlight how caregivers' education, in order to implement care, needs to be also multifaceted, and so has to include theoretical, technical/practical and psychological aspects of care. Besides, several studies have pointed out the importance of technical and personalized training directly at the caregiver's home, or of an online training carried out by psychologists to reduce anxiety. Other studies have demonstrated that psycho-educational interventions of sharing and discussing caregivers' experience can be a valid support (using both a theoretical approach and emotions expressed) for care burden and emotional distress (Cianfrocca et al., 2018). Also, caregivers at risk of burnout can have training and support to help them to enhance their psychological resources and protective factors (like life satisfaction, confidence and resilience), support that can be provided also with the aid of Information and Communications Technologies (Fianco et al., 2015). Barbabella et al. (2016) argue that in the European Union research and projects have in recent years concentrated on the development and testing of new educative and supportive solutions for older citizens' caregivers, especially in terms of psychoeducational and psychotherapeutic Web-based programs.

Awareness on Interpersonal Touch

This paper highlights the benefits of an integration of "awareness on touch" courses or workshops into formal, or more institutional, educational training for caregivers, healthcare and direct care personnel (in all possible formats). However, there are in literature still few experiences describing

---

[13] Social initiatives directed to caregiver education and support are present in the Italian National Health System: https://www.aslroma1.it/caregiver#

such an approach, both in education and in healthcare studies. In fact, we can find more experiences or studies of carers education on touching through a massage technique, rather than an awareness course solely based on physical touch. This is probably because massage has permeated the culture of care; moreover, it is the most represented and studied complementary care practice in scientific literature, therefore it is much easier to promote in institutions and perhaps be accepted by the healthcare and medical staff (Field, 2016).

Collinge, Kahn, Walton, Kozak, Bauer-Wu, Fletcher, Yarnold & Soltysik (2013) argue that integrating touch as routine supportive care for informal caregivers can be useful for both caring relationship actors: patient and relative. Especially in oncology and palliative care fields, studies are showing how family caregivers trained in complementary care can reduce pain and anxiety in cancer patients. Also, hands-on caregiver education for family members can help to build their sense of self-efficacy and empower them with care. Collinge et al. (2013) study consisted of a randomized controlled trial of a multimedia caregiver education program; such a program was a combined intervention with touch and massage designed for family caregivers. The study highlighted caregivers' high degree of satisfaction while becoming more comfortable with touch and massage, thus increasing perceived self-efficacy. Moreover, the caregiver's ability to participate in patients' well-being was improved and so the quality of their relationship. This experience inspired another study, this time involving caregivers and veterans with a cancer diagnosis. In this study, the multimedia caregiver program was used successfully with caregivers who massaged veterans and reported improved well-being (Kozak, Vig, Simons, Eugenio, Collinge & Chapko, 2013).

Education to touch using multimedia devices have been, moreover, designed for carers and relatives of elderly citizens and individuals with dementia in several settings (Tuohy, Graham, Johnson, Tuohy & Burke, 2015). In this experience, a nursing research team has developed an educational DVD, described as an easily accessible resource, consisting of a hand massage sequence showed step by step. Touhy et al. (2015) reported this experience as highly rewarding, easy to replicate and possible object of further studies; since 2012 this DVD has been distributed widely in several institutions, home and community care in Ireland. Some educational interventions depicted scenarios where, once relatives and carers have been introduced to massage and touch technique, they acquired valid support to elderly care and especially for dementia care. The results of a recent meta-analysis of non-pharmacological interventions showed that massage and touch have a statistically significant effect on decreasing symptoms and agitation in dementia, particularly physical aggressive behavior (Suzuki, Tatsumi, Otsuka, Kikuchi, Mizuta, Makino, Kiruto, Fujiwama, Abe, Nagagomi & Hayashi, 2010; Wu, Wang & Wang, 2017).

Palliative care represents another field where special attention has been given to family or caregivers' touch and massage training. A Swedish body of studies (Cronfalk, Strang, Ternestedt & Friedrichsen, 2009; Cronfalk, Ternestedt & Strang, 2010) has been particularly concerned with how to support relatives and family adopting a soft-tissue massage technique training. A one-day course in massage was used to both improve patients' and carers' well-being and also to help the grieving process. However, the studies of experiences exclusively directed to informal caregivers' touch or massage skills and education are still few, whereas this topic has been more represented by nursing literature. It must be said that most of the nursing studies (considering the ethical and ontological premises and differences) showing an education on touch and caring can foresee a possible application also for informal caregivers. In the Ozolins, Hörberg & Dahlberg (2015) research, a "Caring touch course" has been introduced to nurses and applied in residential homes and elderly care; the findings of this qualitative study show that caring touch can have a deep impact on a human being and relieve suffering in a variety of ways. In this last study, touch is described as a powerful caring tool (Ozolins et al., 2015). Another important contribution (already mentioned here) is the research on massage training and nurses' compassion fatigue; in this research, nurses who massaged patients described this experience as highly rewarding (Wilson et al., 2016).

An Italian Experience: Training in Touch for Healthcare Assistants

There have been several experiences in the Italian healthcare system of training events dedicated to direct care personnel (recently in a Hospice and long-term care institution based in Milan); these educational interventions have been created by the nursing directorate as part of implemental projects for the humanization of care. Moreover, they aim to raise awareness on this topic and to support nursing and healthcare personnel that are in direct contact with patients. This training has strong practical implications and thus it is structured as an experiential one/two-day workshop: minimal space is given to philosophical premises about the sense of touch and caring theories (more appropriate instead for courses dedicated to nurses).

A training proposal of this type can only prefer the transmission of knowledge that occurs with learning from experience and reflections on practice. The educational approach chosen refers to the adult learning theories and lifelong learning logic, according to which the trainer is a facilitator who supports caregivers. Therefore, the workshop is focused on proposing participants to safely experience different examples of interpersonal contact occurring in a healthcare setting (through role-playing, everyday scenarios vignettes, experiences of sensory deprivation blindfolded and with earplugs, etc.). These experiences help to elicit group discussion, feelings and memories, with the aid of a facilitator and then to let emerge and identify participants learning needs (for example how to mobilize a patient from bed to chair with a special attention on gestures and touch or how to hold a person's leg in a caring way while performing personal hygiene). At the end of the workshop, a small sequence of soft and gentle massage is shown and, under supervision, participants were encouraged to try to perform it on each other. The participants workshop satisfaction has been very high and from post-training questionnaire reports it emerged that the training on awareness of touch had helped them to improve their practice, to find solutions within caring relationship conflicts, to reflect on the impact of contact within patients' care, and on how to change their caring gestures so as to improve communication. In conclusion, it must be considered that this last experience is different from a multimedia intervention, a web-based program or even a brief massage course, and therefore it needs to be considered the topic of possible future research.

CONCLUSION

The current evidence of caregiving health risks represents a shift of paradigm from only studying the care recipients to a broader perspective in which the caregiver is also included as an object of attention (Cuéllar-Flores, del Pilar Sánchez-López & Santamaría, 2012). The interest in formal or informal caregivers' well-being and psychosocial functioning elicited a research field that highlighted the fragility of this caring position. However, it has been outlined how providing good care to others does not always lead to the caregiver's psychological adjustment, even when he/she possess the appropriate cognitive and affective resources (Cuellar et al., 2012). Nowadays, it seems unrealistic to assume that informal caregiving performed by familial or paid carers is an unskilled job, performed just out of personal vocation or for necessity, or because belonging to a gender, but it is a job that needs support and education. Caregivers spend time with their clients or relatives, in washing, feeding and walking them. Moreover, they have to get into contact with them, to know them (and their families), and to develop a relationship even when the person seems to be cognitively unreachable. The impact of touch, within the caring relationship, might have been underestimated, and a substantial body of research has highlighted how the quality of touch of healthcare professionals can be improved. Besides, integrating massage, gentle and intentional forms of contact in personal comfort care is an opportunity to restore assistance to a more human and welcoming dimension (Connor & Howett, 2009).

During the personal hygiene routine, this special attention to our contact style and gestures, in approaching the intimacy of the other, allows the carer to find and "redefine" the contours of the relational space with the person they are assisting (Prayez & Savatofski, 2009). There are circumstances where caregivers have the chance to transform their daily routine, and from here their gestures, into a meaningful experience and to improve the caring relationship. Although our touch predisposition is influenced by several factors (like our attachment style and developmental history), to touch in a more intentional and caring manner is something that can be taught and learned. In addition, "comfort with touch" studies by Pedrazza et al. (2015; 2018) have shown that healthcare personnel who are less touch-avoidant and more at ease with interpersonal contact, are less exposed to burnout and possess more compassion satisfaction. In fact, recent research has already shown how much the healthcare operator who reflects on contact practices or who uses another way to be in contact with others (such as a simple and gentle massage technique) can experience a reduction of the sense of non-belonging and dissatisfaction (Wilson et al., 2016; Ozolins et al., 2015).

Older citizens are often not touched anymore or perceived as "untouchable" due to isolation, socio-cultural issues or clinical and neurological conditions (such as Dementia, Alzheimer's Disease, etc.). Therefore, to raise awareness and train caregivers about the impact and the quality of their touching style can represent a priority, especially in conditions where there is a high patient/relative dependency and constant care is required for physical comfort and mobilization. Once caregivers have an awareness and are encouraged to reflect on touch, patients will physically and psychologically inevitably benefit from it. The quality and attention to the way a caregiver touches, enhanced and implemented by training, will help to support communication, and also to ameliorate conditions where there is a patient's agitation or anxiety. McFeeters, Pront, Cuthbertson & King (2016) and Kolcaba, Schirm & Steiner (2006) state that the person who perceives to be touched with caring gestures will have an improvement of his/her overall wellbeing and implement the feeling of being taken care of. In this way, the conditions can be created to build, around the patient, a respectful and attentive model of caregiving; a model that can consider the personal uniqueness, expectations, and desires.

In conclusion, I would like to add that, as an experienced nurse, teacher, and researcher in adult education, I have personally witnessed, in many settings, how caregivers' working life can be improved with training (perhaps included into a broader training program) on awareness of interpersonal contact. Furthermore, education on contact focusing on how to touch and how it can become a personal resource to deal with the burden of care, is fundamental for caregivers and, as a natural extension, for the patient's well-being. Taking inspiration from the reflective learning paradigm and recalling the reciprocity of the sense of touch, we can simply state that the act itself of taking care of others is to take care of ourselves; hence, to be aware of our presence and contact abilities, in a caring relationship, renders the overall caring experience a rewarding one. After all, this process represents an expression of the transformative potential of lifelong learning and it can only be found in the hands of caregivers.

REFERENCES

Adelman, R. D., Tmanova, L. L., Delgado, D., Dion, S. & Lachs, M. S. (2014). Caregiver burden: a clinical review. *Journal of American Medical Association*, *311*(10), 1052-1060. doi: 10.1001/ jama.2014.304.

Aksoydan, E., Aytar, A., Blazeviciene, A., van Bruchem-Visser, R. L., Vaskelyte, A., Mattace-Raso, F. & Baskici, C. (2019). Is training for informal caregivers and their older persons helpful? A systematic review. *Archives of gerontology and geriatrics*, *83*, 66-74. doi: 10.1016/j.archger.2019.02.006.

Barbabella, F., Poli, A., Andréasson, F., Salzmann, B., Papa, R., Hanson, E. & Lamura, G. (2016). A web-based psychosocial intervention for family caregivers of older people: results from a mixed-methods study in three European countries. *JMIR research protocols*, *5*(4), e196. doi: 10.2196/resprot.5847.

Benner, P., Tanner, C. A. & Chesla, C. A. (2009). *Expertise in nursing practice: Caring, clinical judgment, and ethics.*: New York, NY: Springer Publishing Company.

Blasdell, N. D. (2017). The meaning of caring in nursing practice. *International Journal of Nursing & Clinical Practices*, *4*(238), 2. doi: 10.15344/2394-4978/2017/238.

Bruni, M. L. & Ugolini, C. (2016). Delegating home care for the elderly to external caregivers? An empirical study on Italian data. *Review of Economics of the Household*, *14*(1), 155-183. doi: 10.1007/s11150-014-9253-x.

Canzan, F., Heilemann, M. V., Saiani, L., Mortari, L. & Ambrosi, E. (2014). Visible and invisible caring in nursing from the perspectives of patients and nurses in the gerontological context. *Scandinavian journal of caring sciences*, *28*(4), 732-740.

Castagnone, E., Salis, E. & Premazzi, V. (2013). *Promoting Integration of Migrant Domestic Workers in Italy*. Geneva: International Labour Organization.

Chang, S. O. (2001). The conceptual structure of physical touch in caring. *Journal of advanced nursing*, *33*(6), 820-827.

Cianfrocca, C., Caponnetto, V., Donati, D., Lancia, L., Tartaglini, D. & Di Stasio, E. (2018). The effects of a multidisciplinary education course on the burden, health literacy and needs of family caregivers. *Applied Nursing Research*, *44*, 100-106.

Cocksedge, S., George, B., Renwick, S. & Chew-Graham, C. A. (2013). Touch in primary care consultations: qualitative investigation of doctors' and patients' perceptions. *British Journal of General Practice*, *63*(609), e283-e290.

Collinge, W., Kahn, J., Walton, T., Kozak, L., Bauer-Wu, S., Fletcher, K. & Soltysik, R. (2013). Touch, Caring, and Cancer: randomized controlled trial of a multimedia caregiver education program. *Supportive Care in Cancer*, *21*(5), 1405-1414.

Connor, A. & Howett, M. (2009). A conceptual model of intentional comfort touch. *Journal of Holistic Nursing*, *27*(2), 127-135.

Cronfalk, B. S., Strang, P., Ternestedt, B. M. & Friedrichsen, M. (2009). The existential experiences of receiving soft tissue massage in palliative home care—an intervention. *Supportive care in cancer*, *17*(9), 1203-1211.

Cronfalk, B. S., Ternestedt, B. M. & Strang, P. (2010). Soft tissue massage: early intervention for relatives whose family members died in palliative cancer care. *Journal of clinical nursing*, *19*(7-8), 1040-1048.

Croy, I., Sehlstedt, I., Wasling, H. B., Ackerley, R. & Olausson, H. (2017). Gentle touch perception: From early childhood to adolescence. *Developmental cognitive neuroscience*, *35*, 81-86. doi: 10.1016/ j.dcn.2017.07.009.

Cuéllar-Flores, I., del Pilar Sánchez-López, M. & Santamaría, P. (2012). Personality and psychological adjustment in formal caregivers. What is best for caring is also the best for caregivers? *Anuario de Psicología*, *42*(2), 151-164.

Da Roit, B. & Le Bihan, B. (2010). Similar and yet so different: cash-for-care in six European countries' long-term care policies. *The Milbank Quarterly*, *88*(3), 286-309.

De Vignemont, F. (2010). Body schema and body image—Pros and cons. *Neuropsychologia*, *48*(3), 669-680.

Di Rosa, M., Barbabella, F., Chiatti, C., Melchiorre, M. G. & Lamura, G. (2013). Private employment of home care workers and use of health services by disabled older people in Italy. *Euroregional Journal of Socio-Economic Analysis*, *1*(1), 33-42.

Eleuteri, S., Bellanti, G. & Falaschi, P. (2016). Hip fracture: preliminary results supporting significant correlations between the psychological wellbeing of patients and their relative caregivers. *Journal of Gerontology & Geriatrics*, *64*, 104-111.

Eleuteri, S., Norton, M. C., Livi, F., Grano, C., Lucidi, F., Violani, C. & Lombardo, C. (2018). *Sleep quality as predictor of BMI in non-depressed caregivers of people with dementia, Eating and Weight Disorders*, *23*(5), 553-560. doi: 10.1007/s40519-018-0560-8.

Estabrooks, C. A. & Morse, J. M. (1992). Toward a theory of touch: the touching process and acquiring a touching style. *Journal of advanced nursing*, *17*(4), 448-456.

Fianco, A., Sartori, R. D., Negri, L., Lorini, S., Valle, G. & Delle Fave, A. (2015). The relationship between burden and well-being among caregivers of Italian people diagnosed with severe neuromotor and cognitive disorders. *Research in Developmental Disabilities*, *39*, 43-54.

Field, T. (2016). Massage therapy research review. *Complementary therapies in clinical practice*, *24*, 19-31.

Fisher, J. D., Rytting, M. & Heslin, R. (1976). Hands touching hands: Affective and evaluative effects of an interpersonal touch. *Sociometry*, *39*(4), 416-421.

Fredriksson, L. (1999). Modes of relating in a caring conversation: a research synthesis on presence, touch and listening. *Journal of advanced nursing*, *30*(5), 1167-1176.

Fugali, E. (2013). Scritto sulla pelle. Le sensazioni localizzate all'origine del sé corporeo nella fenomenologia husserliana. [Written on the Skin. Localized Sensations and the Origins of the Bodily Self in Husserl's Phenomenology]. *Rivista internazionale di Filosofia e Psicologia*, *4*(1), 49-68.

Fulkerson, M. (2014). What Counts as Touch? In D. Stokes, M. Matthen & S. Biggs (Eds.) *Perception and its Modalities*, (pp. 191-204). New York, USA: Oxford University Press.

Gadow, S. (1984). Touch and technology: Two paradigms of patient care. *Journal of Religion and Health*, *23*, 63–69. doi:10.1007/BF00999900.

Gallace, A. & Spence, C. (2010). The science of interpersonal touch: an overview. *Neuroscience & Biobehavioral Reviews*, *34*(2), 246-259.

Gaugler, J. E., Pestka, D. L., Davila, H., Sales, R., Owen, G., Baumgartner, S. A. & Kenney, M. (2018). The complexities of family caregiving at work: A mixed-methods study. *The International Journal of Aging and Human Development*, *87*(4), 347-376. doi.org/10.1177/ 00914150 1775293.

Genet, N., Boerma, W., Kroneman, M., Hutchinson, A. & Saltman, R. B. (2013). Home care across Europe: case studies. *European Observatory on Health Systems and Policies*. Retrieved from: http:// www.euro.who.int/__data/assets/pdf_file/0008/181799/e96757.pdf.

Gitlin, L. N. & Hodgson, N. (2015). Caregivers as therapeutic agents in dementia care: the context of caregiving and the evidence base for interventions. In J. E. Gaugler & R. L. Kane (Eds.) *Family caregiving in the new normal*, (pp. 305-353). San Diego, USA: Elsevier Academic Press.

Gleeson, M. & Timmins, F. (2004). The use of touch to enhance nursing care of older person in long-term mental health care facilities. *Journal of Psychiatric and Mental Health Nursing*, *11*(5), 541-545.

Gleeson, M. & Timmins, F. (2005). A review of the use and clinical effectiveness of touch as a nursing intervention. *Clinical effectiveness in nursing*, *9*(1-2), 69-77.

Grassi, L. (2013). Quam bene vivas referre: curing and caring in psycho-oncology. *Psycho-Oncology*, *22*(8), 1679-1687.

Grousset, S. (2009). Mise au point: Définition et concepts liés au toucher dans les soins [Development: Definition and concepts related to touch in care]. *Soins*, (737), 30-31.

Heidegger, M. (2011). *Essere e tempo* [*Being and Time*] Milan, Italy: Mondadori editions.

Hertenstein, M. J., Keltner, D., App, B., Bulleit, B. A. & Jaskolka, A. R. (2006). Touch communicates distinct emotions. *Emotion*, *6*(3), 528.

Hertenstein, M. J., Verkamp, J. M., Kerestes, A. M. & Holmes, R. M. (2006). The communicative functions of touch in humans, nonhuman primates, and rats: a review and synthesis of the empirical research. *Genetic, social, and general psychology monographs*, *132*(1), 5-94.

Huta, V. (2013). Eudaimonia. In S. A. David, I. Boniwell & A. C. Ayers (Eds.). (2014) *The Oxford handbook of happiness*, (pp. 201-213). New York, NY: Oxford University Press.

Jecker, N. S. & Self, D. J. (1991). Separating care and cure: an analysis of historical and contemporary images of nursing and medicine. *The Journal of Medicine and Philosophy*, *16*(3), 285-306. doi:10.1093/jmp/16.3.285.

Kelly, M. A., Nixon, L., McClurg, C., Scherpbier, A., King, N. & Dornan, T. (2018). Experience of touch in health care: A meta-ethnography across the health care professions. *Qualitative health research*, *28*(2), 200-212.

Kleinman, A. & Van Der Geest, S. (2009). Care in health care. Remaking the moral world of medicine. *Medische Antropologie*, *21*(1), 159.

Kolcaba, K., Schirm, V. & Steiner, R. (2006). Effects of hand massage on comfort of nursing home residents. *Geriatric Nursing*, *27*(2), 85-91.

Kozak, L., Vig, E., Simons, C., Eugenio, E., Collinge, W. & Chapko, M. (2013). A feasibility study of caregiver-provided massage as supportive care for Veterans with cancer. *Journal of Supportive Oncology*, *11*(3), 133-143.DOI: 10.12788/j.suponc.0008.

Kübler-Ross, E. & Kessler, D. (2005). *On grief and grieving: Finding the meaning of grief through the five stages of loss*. New York, NY: Scribner.

Leonard, K. E. & Kalman, M. A. (2015). The meaning of touch to patients undergoing chemotherapy. *Oncology nursing forum*, *42*(5), 517-526.

Lindgren, L., Westling, G., Brulin, C., Lehtipalo, S., Andersson, M. & Nyberg, L. (2012). Pleasant human touch is represented in pregenual anterior cingulate cortex. *Neuroimage*, *59*(4), 3427-3432.

Marzano, M. (2007). *La philosophie du corps*. [*The phylosophie of the body*]. Paris, France: Presses Universitaires de France.

McCann, K. & McKenna, H. P. (1993). An examination of touch between nurses and elderly patients in a continuing care setting in Northern Ireland. *Journal of advanced nursing*, *18*(5), 838-846.

McGlone, F., Vallbo, A. B., Olausson, H., Loken, L. & Wessberg, J. (2007). Discriminative touch and emotional touch. *Canadian Journal of Experimental Psychology/Revue Canadienne de psychologie expérimentale*, *61*(3), 173.

McGlone, F., Wessberg, J. & Olausson, H. (2014). Discriminative and affective touch: sensing and feeling. *Neuron*, *82*(4), 737-755.

McFeeters, S., Pront, L., Cuthbertson, L. & King, L. (2016). Massage, a complementary therapy effectively promoting the health and well-being of older people in residential care settings: a review of the literature. *International journal of older people nursing*, *11*(4), 266-283.

Merleau-Ponty, M. (2013). *Phenomenology of perception*. Abingdon, UK: Routledge.

Montagu, A. (1971). *Touching: the human significance of the skin*. New York, NY: Harper & Row.

Moroni, L., Sguazzin, C., Filipponi, L., Bruletti, G., Callegari, S., Galante, E. & Bertolotti, G. (2008). Caregiver Need Assessment: uno strumento di analisi dei bisogni del caregiver. [Caregiver Need Assessment: A

Questionnaire For Caregiver Demand]. *Giornale Italiano di Medicina del Lavoro e Ergonomia*, *30*(3), 19-23.

Morrison, I., Löken, L. S. & Olausson, H. (2010). The skin as a social organ. *Experimental Brain Research*, *204*, 305–314. doi.org/10.1007/ s00221-009-2007-y.

Mortari, L. (2004). Educating to care. *Canadian Journal of Environmental Education*, *9*(1), 109-122.

Mortari, L. & Saiani, L. (2014). *Gestures and thoughts of caring: A theory of caring from the voices of nurses*. New York, NY McGraw-Hill Education.

Nobili, G., Massaia, M., Isaia, G., Cappa, G., Pilon, S., Mondino, S. & Isaia, G. C. (2011). Valutazione dei bisogni del caregiver di pazienti affetti da demenza: esperienza in una unità di valutazione Alzheimer. *Giornale di Gerontologia*, [Evaluation of the needs of caregivers for patients with Alzheimer's disease: experience in a memory clinic]., *59*(2), 71-74.

Nussbaum, M. C. (2001) *L'intelligenza delle Emozioni*. [*Upheavals of Thought: The Intelligence of Emotions*]. Bologna, Italy: Il Mulino edizioni.

Ogden, P., Minton, K. & Pain, C. (2006). *Trauma and the body: A sensorimotor approach to psychotherapy*. New York, NY: Norton Editions.

Olausson, H., Cole, J., Rylander, K., McGlone, F., Lamarre, Y., Wallin, B. G. & Vallbo, Å. (2008). Functional role of unmyelinated tactile afferents in human hairy skin: sympathetic response and perceptual localization. *Experimental brain research*, *184*(1), 135-140.

Ozolins, L. L., Hörberg, U. & Dahlberg, K. (2015). Caring touch–patients' experiences in an anthroposophic clinical context. *Scandinavian journal of caring sciences*, *29*(4), 834-842.

Paniccia, R. M., Giovagnoli, F. & Caputo, A. (2015). In-home elder care. The case of Italy: The badante. *Rivista di Psicologia Clinica*, (2), 60-83. doi: 10.14645/RPC.2014.2.506.

Pedrazza, M., Minuzzo, S., Berlanda, S. & Trifiletti, E. (2015). Nurses' comfort with touch and workplace well-being. *Western journal of nursing research*, *37*(6), 781-798.

Pedrazza, M., Berlanda, S., Trifiletti, E. & Minuzzo, S. (2018). Variables of individual difference and the experience of touch in nursing. *Western journal of nursing research*, *40*(11), 1614-1637.

Pennacchini, M., Petriccione, A., Sisto, A., Di, I. L., Santo Di, S. & Tartaglini, D. (2014). Family caregiver education: an Italian experience. *La Clinica terapeutica*, *165*(5), e357-61. doi:10.7417/ T.2014.1763.

Prayez, P. & Savatofski, J. (2009). *Le toucher apprivoisé (3e ed.)*. [*The domesticated touch, 3rd eds*]. Rueil-Malmaison, France: Éditions Lamarre.

Reich, W. T. (1995). History of the Notion of Care. In Reich, W. T. *Encyclopedia of Bioethics* (2nd edn), (pp. 319-331). New York: Simon & Schuster Macmillan.

Reich, W. T. (2012). From ancient consolation and negative care to modern empathy and the neurosciences. *Theoretical medicine and bioethics*, *33*(1), 25-32.

Rodriguez, D. L. & Barbagallo, M. (2012). Long-Term Care nell'Italia che Invecchia. [Long term care in Ageing Italy]. *Giornale di Gerontologia*, *60*(60), 251-254.

Routasalo, P. (1999). Physical touch in nursing studies: a literature review. *Journal of Advanced Nursing*, *30*(4), 843-850.

Routasalo, P. & Isola, A. (1998). Touching by skilled nurses in elderly nursing care. *Scandinavian journal of caring sciences*, *12*(3), 170-178.

Salzmann-Erikson, M. & Eriksson, H. (2005). Encountering touch: A path to affinity in psychiatric care. *Issues in mental health nursing*, *26*(8), 843-852.

Sardadvar, K., Hohnen, P., Kuemmerling, A., McClelland, C., Naujaniene, R. & Villosio, C. (2012). Underpaid, Overworked, but Happy? Ambiguous Experiences and Processes of Vulnerabilisation in Domiciliary Elderly Care. *E-Journal of International and Comparative Labour Studies*, *1*(3-4), 139-168.

Serino, A., & Haggard, P. (2010). Touch and the body. *Neuroscience & Biobehavioral Reviews*, *34*(2), 224-236.

Schuengel, C., Kef, S., Damen, S. & Worm, M. (2010). 'People who need people': attachment and professional caregiving. *Journal of Intellectual Disability Research*, *54*, 38-47.

Spasova, S., Baeten, R., Coster, S., Ghailani, D., Peña-Casas, R. & Vanhercke, B. (2018). Challenges in long-term care in Europe. *A study of national policies, European Social Policy Network (ESPN).* Brussels: European Commission.

Suanet, B., van Groenou, M. B. & Van Tilburg, T. (2012). Informal and formal home-care use among older adults in Europe: can cross-national differences be explained by societal context and composition? *Ageing & Society*, *32*(3), 491-515.

Suzuki, M., Tatsumi, A., Otsuka, T., Kikuchi, K., Mizuta, A., Makino, K. & Hayashi, T. (2010). Physical and psychological effects of 6-week tactile massage on elderly patients with severe dementia. *American Journal of Alzheimer's Disease & Other Dementias*, *25*(8), 680-686. doi.org/ 10.1177%2F1533317510386215.

Tan, J. Y., Molassiotis, A., Lloyd-Williams, M. & Yorke, J. (2018). Burden, emotional distress and quality of life among informal caregivers of lung cancer patients: An exploratory study. *European journal of cancer care*, *27*(1), e12691. doi:10.1111/ecc.12691.

Tuohy, D., Graham, M. M., Johnson, K., Tuohy, T. & Burke, K. (2015). Developing an educational DVD on the use of hand massage in the care of people with dementia: An innovation. *Nurse education in practice*, *15*(4), 299-303.

Wehrle, M. (2018). Being a body and having a body. The twofold temporality of embodied intentionality. *Phenomenology and the Cognitive Sciences*, *07*, 1-23. doi:10.1007/s11097-019-09610-z.

Weiss, S. J. & Niemann, S. K. (2011). Measurement of touch behavior In M. J. Hertenstein & S. J. Weiss (Eds) *The handbook of touch: Neuroscience, Behavioral, and Health Perspectives*, (pp. 245-270). New York, NY: Springer.

Williams, A. M. (2018). Education, training, and mentorship of caregivers of Canadians experiencing a life-limiting illness. *Journal of palliative medicine*, *21*(S1), S-45. doi: 10.1089/jpm.2017.0393.

Wilson, M., Gettel, V., Walsh, J. & Esquenazi, S. (2016). Caring Compassionately for Hospitalized Patients: Can Nurse-Delivered Massage Address Compassion Fatigue? *International Journal of Human Caring*, *20*(3), 146-154.

Wu, J., Wang, Y. & Wang, Z. (2017). The effectiveness of massage and touch on behavioural and psychological symptoms of dementia: A quantitative systematic review and meta-analysis. *Journal of advanced nursing*, *73*(10), 2283-2295.

Yuen, E. Y., Knight, T., Ricciardelli, L. A. & Burney, S. (2018). Health literacy of caregivers of adult care recipients: A systematic scoping review. *Health & social care in the community*, *26*(2), e191-e206.

In: Caregiving
Editor: Stefano Eleuteri

ISBN: 978-1-53616-889-1

Chapter 6

SOCIO-ECONOMIC STATUS OF CAREGIVERS OF HEMODIALYSIS PATIENTS

Georgia Gerogianni[1] and Eirini Grapsa[2]
[1]Department of Nursing, University of West Attica, Athens, Greece
[2]Department of Nephrology, 'Aretaieio' Hospital, National and Kapodistrian University of Athens, Athens, Greece

ABSTRACT

Family caregivers play an important role in the support of dialysis people since they have poor physical status and difficulty in looking after themselves. Caregivers accompany patients to renal unit, manage complications of dialysis treatment, prepare patients' diet and help them with home activities.

However, family carers usually have physical and psychological burden, while they are disappointed due to the problems derived from this therapy. They usually have increased levels of anxiety and depression due to their bad financial situation, the severity of patients' pain, the long duration of hemodialysis and the old patient's age.

Additionally, those who live with dialysis people have limitations in their personal and social activities, while they often face difficulties with their job in order to look after their loved persons. Moreover, many caregivers feel anxiety about home haemodialysis, since they have to learn about new technologies and management of safety issues.

Thus, renal professionals need to provide family caregivers with effecting information and psychological support in order to improve their psychological status and the quality of their life.

Keywords: hemodialysis, family caregivers, dialysis patients, socio-economic status

INTRODUCTION

Hemodialysis includes a variety of complications and restrictions which negatively affect patients' life and increase their dependency on their family members (Gilbertson et al., 2019). Dialysis patients are usually old and have a variety of disabilities including decline in cognitive function (Bayoumi, 2014), sleep disorders, malnutrition (Sattar, Khan, Ahmad, & Danish, 2016), fatigue, infertility, sexual dysfunctions, problems with bones, anaemia, cardiovascular disorders (Shahgholian & Yousefi, 2015).

Family caregivers play an important role in the support of these individuals since they have poor physical well-being and difficulty in looking after themselves. Caregivers accompany patients to renal unit, prevent complications of hemodialysis, prepare patients' diet (Grapsa & Gerogianni, 2018), remind them about their medication, arrange appointments with health professionals and help them with personal hygiene (Bawazier, Stanley, Sianipar, & Suhardjono, 2018). However, sometimes family caregivers must decide whether their patients will interrupt dialysis treatment or will go to a hospice (Grapsa & Gerogianni, 2018).

It is important to note that living with dialysis patients is stressful for caregivers due to repeated patients' hospitalizations (Rajkhowa, 2019). Caregivers of dialysis patients experience high rates of depression, anxiety, fatigue, social isolation, physical, emotional, and financial stress, which leads to higher mortality rates. The long-term provision of care leads to changes in caregivers' life and to limited social activities, since they spend about 3 days a week to accompany their patients to hemodialysis centre (Shdaifat & Manaf, 2012).

Additionally, caregivers of dialysis patients have increased risk for anxiety and depression due to patients' co-morbid diseases, frequent admissions to hospital, chronic pain, sleep disorders, increased sexual problems, uremic symptoms and non-adherence to therapy (Gerogianni, Kouzoupis, & Grapsa, 2018 a; Gerogianni, Lianos, Kouzoupis, Polikandrioti, ·& Grapsa, 2018 b).

Moreover, Gerogianni et al. (2019), in a cross-sectional study with 414 pairs of patients and caregivers, found a significant relation between the rates of anxiety and depression among patients and carers. More specifically, carers had high rates of anxiety and depression when their patients had high rates of anxiety and depression as well.

It has been found that caregivers of dialysis patients have lower quality of life than carers of patients with other chronic diseases. Additionally, caregivers with more health problems experience heavier burden (Gilbertson et al., 2019) while their burden is higher when patients are dependent on them for their self-care needs (Cagan et al., 2018; Hawamdeh, Almari, Almutairi, & Dator, 2017).

Changes in carers' plans about future frequently lead to emotional burden (Gerogianni et al., 2019a), due to physical and psychological problems of their patients and the continuous provision of care. Thus, they experience tension and feelings of hopelessness since they must undertake a variety of activities and responsibilities without the proper experience, leading them to meet patients' needs over their own (Rajkhowa et al., 2019).

Socio-Economic Status of Caregivers

Informal caregivers have to cope with physical, psychological and social stressors that affect their health conditions and quality of life negatively (Eleuteri, Bellanti & Falaschi, 2016). Families of dialysis patients experience increased stress since kidney disease requires a long-term treatment, frequent visits to the hospital, high financial cost and changes in family roles. The permanent stress of caregivers may lead to clinical depression when it is not recognized and managed appropriately (Hawamdeh et al., 2017). Informal caregivers have been repeatedly acknowledged as a model of chronic stress, due to the high level of daily stress that caregivers experience (Eleuteri et al., 2018).

Saeed, Ahmad, Shakoor, Ghafoor, & Kanwal, (2012) found that 33.4% of carers had moderate to severe depression due to poor financial situation. Caregivers with poor financial condition had higher burden of care and increased health problems since they were unable to afford expenses of patients' care.

Additionally, female caregivers and those with 3 or more children were found to have high burden due to their increased responsibilities in family and children care (Cagan et al., 2018). Women are particularly vulnerable to the provision of care since they usually live with their patients and provide care for many hours (Gerogianni & Grapsa, 2018). Similarly, parents, spouses and adult children had higher caregiver burden than other family members (Zhang et al., 2016). However, the spousal relationship may be protective for dialysis patients (Gilbertson et al., 2019).

Metzelthin et al. (2017) found that carers' burden was negatively affected by patients' comorbid diseases, increased rates of disabilities, provision of care for many hours and living together with patients. In another research emerged that caregivers of both genders, but particularly women, who live with patients, have higher levels of depression than carers who do not live with their patients (Caputo et al., 2016).

It was found that carers above 40 years old, having less than 10 years of academic education and receiving less social support had higher burden. Carers' burden had a strong association with their responsibilities since they were not professionals and frequently had inadequate knowledge about kidney failure (Shakya, Tuladhar, & Poudel, 2017). However, carers with higher level of academic education had less self-perceived burden in comparison to those with lower level of education (Zhang et al., 2016).

Caregivers' Age

The increased age of dialysis patients is frequently associated with increased age of their caregivers (Gilbertson et al., 2019), who have similar physical and psychological problems (Shakya, Tuladhar, & Poudel, 2017) and a reduction of the quality of their life (Shdaifat & Manaf, 2012), since they suffer from health problems and have limited social life (Pinquart & Sörensen, 2011).

Limitation in Social Activities

Zhang et al. (2016) found that caregivers who had to provide full time care every day had higher rates of stress than those who provided part time care. Thus, when caregivers have their own job, apart from their caregiving role, it can protect them from depression (Gilbertson et al., 2019). It is important to note that spouses of patients on hemodialysis participate in limited social activities due to their increased workload (Gerogianni & Grapsa, 2018).

Difficulties with Job

Patients are usually unable to work after the beginning of haemodialysis which leads to changes of roles into the family and creates negative emotions and psychological distress between patients and their spouses (Cukor et al., 2007; Gerogianni & Grapsa, 2018). They often have problems with work, since they reduce their working hours or early retired in order to provide care to their patients (Gerogianni & Grapsa, 2018). Alnazly (2016) found that 30% of caregivers were unemployed since they used to spend 50 hours a week for provision of care, while they postponed their education, which had a negative effect on their career and their economic condition. Additionally, caregivers of a middle age are usually concerned because they miss workdays and are less productive due to the provision of care (Bayoumi, 2014).

Caregivers' Anxiety about Home Hemodialysis

Many patients receive home hemodialysis treatment which results in better quality of patients' life. However, it leads to increased caregivers' responsibilities and increased burden for caregivers. Walker et al. (2016) found that caregivers with low socio- economic status were concerned about the choice of home hemodialysis due to the additional cost of this treatment modality. They were unable to afford the cost of dialysis at home, such us electricity, water supplies, medical equipment and changes at home. They regarded home hemodialysis as very expensive, which imposed a financial burden to the family and led to increase of stress and pressure on both patients and caregivers.

Support Interventions to Caregivers

The Role of Renal Staff

There is a need for investigation of caregivers' needs and the development of health-promoting and support programs (Rajkhowa, 2019). More specifically, clinical nurses should early assess caregivers' burden, and aid those with inadequate social support. Furthermore, a caregiver support programme should be applied in order to guide management of care at home, provide psychological counselling to caregivers and improve their mental health. Renal nurses need to pay attention on the provision of help to family members in order to adjust to the chronic disease and effectively support their patients. This can be facilitated by the responsibility of health care team to meet patient's overall needs (Salehitali, Ahmadi, Zarea, Fereidooni-Moghadam, 2018).

When caregivers accompany their patients to renal unit, appropriate attention to caregivers' needs by the health care team have positive effects on caregiver's psychological status. Additionally, dialysis nurses need to undertake responsibilities towards the patient based on a defined job description, which can help caregivers feel confidence about renal professionals, while they feel there is no need to be present at the renal unit to take care of their patients which helps them reduce the burden of care (Salehitali et al., 2018).

Additionally, caregivers should have the ability to take part in the care process of their patients in order to have a better feeling of care. Nurses need to pay attention to meet mental and psychological needs of patients and their caregivers. Good nurses are those who can provide comfort, safety, and well-being for patients and their family caregivers, paying attention to patients' body, mind, and soul. The appropriate responsiveness of health care team to patients helps caregivers to feel a sense of hope about patient's health (Salehitali et al., 2018).

Cognitive Behavioural Therapy

Cognitive behavioural therapy is a psychotherapeutic process which can reduce anxiety and depressive symptoms in carers of dialysis people, since it helps people change their negative beliefs and gain control over them (Gerogianni, Babatsikou, Polikandrioti, & Grapsa, 2019 b; Duarte, Miyazaki, Blay, & Sesso, 2009) Cognitive behavioural therapy includes different methods, such as relaxation, cognitive restructuring and exposure which can be applied at an individual basis or in groups (Wolgensinger, 2015).

Physical Exercise

A regular exercise can reduce anxiety and depressive symptoms, since it stimulates the brain to produce endorphins and makes individuals feel happy and relaxed (Chiang, Livneh, Yen, Li, & Tsai, 2013). Exercise activities reduce fatigue and pain in musculoskeletal system (Dziubek et al., 2016), increases strength of muscles, while it improves physical and mental status (Mafra & Fouque, 2014).

Social Support

Social support can improve caregivers' self esteem (Grigoriou et al., 2015) and lead to a reduction of anxiety and depressive symptoms (Radwan et al. 2013). Carayanni et al. (2012) who investigated depressive symptoms among 360 older people in Greece found that meeting friends help people reduce their anxiety, while going on trips and going to church every week protect people from depression. People with higher levels of religiosity and spirituality usually receive better social support via their large social network (Lucchetti et al., 2010).

Additionally, hemodialysis caregivers can participate in network support groups and receive online self- help therapy by renal professionals and the appropriate information concerning dialysis patients' care (Hudson et al., 2016).

Conclusion

Family caregivers play a significant role in the support of people undergoing hemodialysis since they can help them with different activities. However, they frequently have physical and psychological burden and increased rates of depression and anxiety due to restrictions of hemodialysis on their daily life. Thus, renal professionals can provide them with effecting information and psychological support in order to improve their psychosocial well-being.

REFERENCES

Alnazly, E. (2016). Burden and coping strategies among Jordanian caregivers of patients undergoing hemodialysis. *Hemodialysis International*, 20, 84-93. doi: 10.1111/hdi.12318.

Bawazier, L., Stanley, I., Sianipar, W., & Suhardjono, S. (2018). Anxiety and depression among caregivers of hemodialysis patients at the Indonesian national referral hospital. *Medical Journal of Indonesia*, 27, 271-8. doi: https://doi.org/10.13181/mji.v27i4.2999.

Bayoumi, M. (2014). Subjective Burden on Family Carers of Hemodialysis Patients. *Open Journal of Nephrology*, 4, 79-85. doi: 10.4236/ojneph. 2014.42011.

Cagan, O., Unsal, A., Celik, N., Ture, Yilmaz, A. T., Culha, I., & Eren, H. K. (2018). Care burden of caregivers of hemodialysis patients and related factors. *International Journal of Caring Sciences*, 11 (1), 279-284.

Caputo, J., Pavalko, E., & Hardy, M. (2016). The long-term effects of caregiving on women's health and mortality. *Journal of Marriage and Family*, 78 (5), 1382-1398. doi: 10.1111/ jomf.12332.

Carayanni, V., Stylianopoulou, C., Koulierakis, G., Babatsikou, F., & Koutis, C. (2012). Sex differences in depression among older adults: are older women more vulnerable than men in social risk factors? The case of open care centers for older people in Greece. *European Journal of Ageing*, 9 (2), 177-186. doi:10.1007/s1043 3-012-0216-x.

Chiang, H., Livneh, H., Yen, M., Li, T., & Tsai, T. (2013). Prevalence and correlates of depression among chronic kidney disease patients in Taiwan. *BMC Nephrology*, 14: 1-8. doi: 10.1186/1471-2369-14-78.

Cukor, D., Cohen, S., Peterson, R., & Kimmel, P. (2007). Psychosocial aspects of chronic disease: ESRD as a paradigmatic Illness. *Journal of the American Society of Nephrology*, 18, 3042-3055. doi: https://doi. org/10.1681/ASN.2007030345.

Duarte, P., Miyazaki, M., Blay, S., & Sesso, R. (2009). Cognitive-behavioral group therapy is an effective treatment for major depression in hemodialysis patients. *Kidney International*, 76, 414-421. doi: 10. 1038/ki.2009.156.

Dziubek, W., Kowalska, J., Kusztal, M., Rogowski, Ł., Gołębiowski, T., Nikifur, M., ... Woźniewski, M. (2016). The level of anxiety and depression in dialysis patients undertaking regular physical exercise training - a preliminary study. *Kidney Blood Pressure Research*, 4, 86-98. doi: 10.1159/00036 8548.

Eleuteri S., Bellanti G., & Falaschi P., (2016). Hip fracture: preliminary results supporting significant correlations between the psychological wellbeing of patients and their relative caregivers, *Journal of Gerontology & Geriatrics*, 64, 104-111.

Eleuteri, S., Norton, M. C., Livi, F., Grano, C., Lucidi, F., Violani, C., ... Lombardo, C. (2018) Sleep quality as predictor of BMI in non-depressed caregivers of people with dementia, *Eating and Weight Disorders*, 23(5), 553-560.

Gerogianni, G., Babatsikou, F., Polikandrioti, M., & Grapsa, E. (2019b). Management of anxiety and depression in haemodialysis patients: The role of non pharmacological methods. *International Urology and Nephrology*, 51, 113-118. doi: 10.1007/s11255-018-2022-7.

Gerogianni, G., Kouzoupis, A., & Grapsa, E. (2018a). A holistic approach to factors affecting depression in haemodialysis patients. *International Urology and Nephrology*, 50: 1467-1476. https://doi.org/10.1007/s 11255-018-1891-0.

Gerogianni, G., Lianos, E., Kouzoupis, A., Polikandrioti, M.,·& Grapsa, E. (2018b). The role of socio-demographic factors in depression and anxiety of patients on hemodialysis: an observational cross-sectional study. *International Urology and Nephrology*, 50 (1), 143-154. doi: 10. 1007/s11255-017-1738-0.

Gerogianni, G., Polikandrioti, M., Babatsikou, F., Zyga, S., Alikari, V., Vasilopoulos, G., ... Grapsa, E. (2019a). Anxiety-Depression of Dialysis Patients and Their Caregivers. *Medicina* (Kaunas), 55 (5), E168. doi: 10.3390/medicina55050168.

Gilbertson, E., Krishnasamy, R., Foote, C., Kennard, A., Jardine, M., & Gray, N. (2019). Burden of care and quality of life among caregivers for adults receiving maintenance dialysis: A systematic review. *American Journal of Kidney Diseases*, 73 (3), 332-343. doi: 10. 1053/j.ajkd. 2018.09.006.

Grapsa E, & Gerogianni G. (2018). Caregivers of patients on haemodialysis. In: M. Mollaoglu (Ed). *Caregiving and Home Care*. Retrieved from: http://www.intechopen.com/books/caregiving-and-home-care. doi: 10. 5772/intechopen.72400.

Grigoriou, S., Karatzaferi, C., & Sakkas, G. (2015). Pharmacological and non-pharmacological treatment options for depression and depressive symptoms in haemodialysis patients. *Health Psychology Research*, 3, 1811. doi: 10.4081/hpr.2015.1811.

Hawamdeh, S., Almari, A. M., Almutairi, A. S., & Dator, W. L. (2017). Determinants and prevalence of depression in patients with chronic renal disease, and their caregivers. *International Journal of Nephrology and Renovascular Disease*, 10, 183-189. doi: https://doi. org/10.2147/ IJNRD.S139652.

Hudson, J., Moss-Morris, R., Game, D., Carroll, A., McCrone, P., Hotopf, M., Yardley, L., Chilcot, J. (2016). Improving distress in dialysis (iDiD): a feasibility two-arm parallel randomised controlled trial of an online cognitive behavioural therapy intervention with and without therapist-led telephone support for psychological distress in patients undergoing haemodialysis. *BMJ Open*, 6, e011286. https://doi.org/10. 1136/bmjop en-2016-01128 6.

Lucchetti, G., Camargo de Almeida, L., & Granero, A. (2010). Spirituality for dialysis patients: should the nephrologist address? *Brazilian Journal of Nephrology*, 32 (1), 126-130. http://dx.doi.org/10.1590/S 0101-28002010000100020.

Mafra, D., & Fouque, D. (2014). Lower physical activity and depression are associated with hospitalization and shorter survival in CKD. *Clinical Journal of the American Society of Nephrology*, 9 (10), 1669-1670. doi: 10.2215/CJN.08400 814.

Metzelthin, S., Verbakel, E., Veenstra, M., Exel, J., Ambergen, A., & Kempen, G. (2017). Positive and negative outcomes of informal caregiving at home and in institutionalised long-term care: A cross-sectional study. *BMC Geriatrics*, 17, 232. doi: 10.1186/s12877-017-0620-3.

Pinquart, M., & Sörensen, S. (2011). Spouses, adult children, and children-in-law as caregivers of older adults: A meta-analytic comparison. *Psychology and Aging*, 26 (1), 1-14. doi: 10.1037/a0021863.

Radwan, D., Sany, D., Elmissiry, A., Shahawy, Y., Fekry, W. (2013). Screening for depression and associated risk factors among Egyptian end-stage renal disease patients on haemodialysis. *Middle East Current Psychiatry*, 20, 183-190. doi: 10.1097/01.XME.00004 33782. 59658. a3.

Rajkhowa, R. (2019). Experiences and difficulties faced by family caregivers of hemodialysis patients in Ranchi, Jharkhand. *International Journal of Research in Engineering, Science and Management*, 2, 40-42.

Rutkowski, B., & Rychlik, I. (2011). Daily haemodialysis and caregiver burden. *Nephrology Dialysis Transplantation*, 26, 2074-2076. doi: 10. 1093/ndt/gfr298.

Saeed, Z., Ahmad, A. M., Shakoor, A., Ghafoor, F., & Kanwal, S. (2012). Depression in patients on hemodialysis and their caregivers. *Saudi Journal of Kidney Disease and Transplantation*, 3 (5), 946-52. doi: 10. 4103/1319-2442.100869.

Salehitali, S., Ahmadi, F., Zarea, K., Fereidooni-Moghadam, M. (2018). The role of heath team in coping process of family caregivers with patients under hemodialysis: a qualitative study. *Jundishapur Journal of Chronic Disease Care*, 7 (1): e63304. doi: 10.5812/jjcdc.63304.

Sattar, S., Khan, N., Ahmad, F., & Danish, S. (2016). Post- dialysis effects in patients on haemodialysis. *Journal of Pakistan Medical Association*, 66 (6), 781-8.

Shahgholian, N., & Yousefi, H. (2015). Supporting hemodialysis patients: A phenomenological study. *Iranian Journal of Nursing and Midwifery Research*, 20 (5): 626-633. doi: 10.4103/1735-9066.164514.

Shakya, D., Tuladhar, J., & Poudel, S. (2017). Burden and Depression among Caregivers of Hemodialysis Patients. *Journal of Palliative and Medical Care*, 4 (1), 1-6. doi: 10.15226/2374-8362/4/1/00131.

Shdaifat, E., & Manaf, M. (2012). Quality of Life of Caregivers and Patients Undergoing Haemodialysis at Ministry of Health, Jordan. *International Journal of Applied Science and Technology*, 2 (3), 75-85.

Walker, R., Howard, K., Tong, A., Palmer, S., Marshall, M., & Morton, R. (2016). The economic considerations of patients and caregivers in choice of dialysis modality. *Hemodialysis International*, 20, 634-642. doi: 10.1111/hdi.12424.

Wolgensinger, L. (2015). Cognitive behavioral group therapy for anxiety: recent developments. *Dialogues in Clinical Neuroscience*, 17, 347-351.

Zhang, R., Cui, X., Zhuang, H., Xie, W., lu, L., Liu, Y., & Zheng, F. (2016). The Burden for caring patients on maintenance hemodialysis is influenced by social and demographic factors. *General Medicine* (Los Angeles), 4, 6. doi: 10.4172/2327-5146.1000281.

In: Caregiving
Editor: Stefano Eleuteri
ISBN: 978-1-53616-889-1

Chapter 7

Caregiving Partners with Autoimmune Rheumatic Diseases: Psychological, Relational and Sexual Impact

***Stefano Eleuteri*[1,*], *Roberta Rossi*[2] *and Chiara Simonelli*[3]**
[1]Department of Psychology, Sapienza University of Rome, Rome, Italy
[2]Institute of Clinical Sexology, Rome
[3]Department of Dynamic and Clinic Psychology
Sapienza University of Rome, Rome, Italy

Abstract

Autoimmune diseases form a range of disorders from organ-specific to systemic disorders with multi-organ involvement. Rheumatic diseases touch all aspects of life and this includes, of course, the partner, with an impact on the relationship, on sexuality and reproduction. The aim of this chapter is to analyze the implications of caregiving a partner with an

* Corresponding Author's Email: stefano.eleuteri@uniroma1.it.

autoimmune rheumatic disease. Diseases will be separately studied, and a final recommendation will be included. Many factors connected to rheumatic autoimmune diseases may cause these patients to become dependent on other people. Increased knowledge and awareness of rheumatologists, nurses, and care providers about physical, sexual, and psychological aspects of care plays an important role in improved management of these patients.

Most patients with sexual dysfunction rarely talked about sexual complaints with their rheumatologist. The sexual health of patients with rheumatic diseases is often neglected, with the possibility for both patients and medical doctors to find it difficult to discuss about sex, in part also because effective treatment options are not still available.

Sexuality is influenced by physical and psychological consequences of rheumatic diseases, like depression, anxiety, negative body image, reduced sexual drive, hormonal imbalance, pain, fatigue, stiffness, functional impairment and side effects from treatments.

The common problem is communication, so an open conversation including inquiry about sexuality in routine care is the first step to improve the situation. To allow the patients to present problems and concerns without embarrassment is also important. After an open discussion is achieved, the treatment will depend on the specific patient's symptoms. However, there are some general recommendations including: discussion of the problems with the partner, principally about the partner's fear in causing pain or distress during sexual intercourse; exploring different positions; using analgesic drugs, heat, and muscle relaxants before sexual activity in order to decrease pain; exploring alternative methods of sexual expression; and physiotherapy.

A multidisciplinary approach is therefore essential, in order to provide prevention and care for their sexual life, providing a better quality of life both for these patients and their partners.

1. INTRODUCTION

Autoimmune diseases form a range of disorders from organ-specific (e.g., Hashimoto's thyroiditis) to systemic disorders with multi-organ involvement. Disorders that mainly, but not exclusively, affect joints and muscles are grouped together as autoimmune rheumatic diseases, and include rheumatoid arthritis, systemic lupus erythematosus, primary Sjögren's syndrome, systemic sclerosis (scleroderma), idiopathic inflammatory myositis, and the systemic vasculitides (Goldblatt & O'Neill,

2013). Literature has shown that some of these disorders may have an impact on quality of life including sexuality in patients, with different psychological, relational and sexual impact on the couple. Sexuality has a significant place in human life and remains important for both men and women despite the aging factor (Pirildar, Müezzinoğlu, & Pirildar, 2004; Eleuteri, Rossi, & Simonelli, 2019; Træen et al., 2019). Rheumatic diseases touch all aspects of life and this includes, of course, the partner, with an impact on the relationship, on sexuality and reproduction (Østensen, 2009; 2017). The aim of this chapter is to analyze the implications of caregiving a partner with an autoimmune rheumatic disease. Diseases will be separately studied, and a final recommendation will be included.

2. Autoimmune Rheumatic Diseases and Impact on Sexuality

2.1. Rheumatoid Arthritis

Rheumatoid arthritis (RA) is a chronic, multisystemic, inflammatory and autoimmune disease with unknown etiology (Carmona, Cross, Williams, Lassere, & March, 2010; Zhang et al., 2018). It is also defined as a synovial disease, which can also affect other organs and systems. It is a progressive disease, characterized by immune-driven chronic inflammation and a variable course involving exacerbations and remissions of disease activity (Jacobi et al., 2003; Coskun, Coskun, Atis, Ergenekon, & Dilek, 2013). The progressive character of RA, with physiological and anatomical impairments, causes irreversible joint damage that results in minor to severe disability and leads to consequences for physical, social and psychological functioning, resulting in decreased general life quality in most patients (Klippel, 1998; Lipsky, 2005; Joseffson & Gard, 2012).

Follow-up studies among RA patients showed that, after 10 years of follow-up, about 20% of the patients had no or minor disabilities, most of the patients were moderately disabled, and about 10% of the patients suffered from severe disablement (Lindqvist, Saxne, Geborek, & Eberhardt, 2002).

The physical impairments and disabilities of patients with RA often impede the performance of activities of daily living (ADL), resulting in the use of a wide variety of health-care services (Jacobi, Triemstra, Rupp, Dinant, & Van Den Bos, 2001).

Additionally, many RA patients need care and help at home, which is mostly provided by informal caregivers. The slow, progressive nature of the disease creates long-term dependency on family and friends. Spouses or partners are expected to bear a large proportion of the burden of caregiving (Revenson & Majerovitz, 1991).

RA inevitably leads to various degrees of disability and it has a profound impact on patient's life regarding social, economic, psychological and sexual aspects (Ehrlich, 1983). In RA patients, diminished sexual motivation, competence and expression could lead to marital unhappiness (Blake, Maisiak, Koplan, Alarcón, & Brown, 1988; Yoshino & Uchida, 1981; Frikha et al., 2011), which may even result in divorce and termination of the relationships when sexual functionality becomes difficult or impossible. Although sexual dysfunction is a significant problem in RA, there is inadequate information about this condition possibly because both patients and physicians avoid talking about sexual issues (Blake et al., 1988; Abdel-Nasser & Ali, 2006; Tavares Queiroz de Almeidaa, de Castro Ferreirac, Shu Kurizkyb, Feitosa Munizd, & da Motab; 2015).

The reasons for disturbances of sexual function and reproduction are multifactorial and comprise disease-related factors as well as therapy.

It can occur before, during and after sexual activities, and can affect sexual health in different perspectives (Tristano, 2014). Physical problems, emotional problems and difficulties of partnership arising from disease related stress contribute to a less active and often lessen joyable sex life (Panush, Mihailescu, Gornisiewicz, & Sutaria, 2000; Aras et al., 2013).

Women with RA suffer from pain, restricted joint movements and fatigue; also probably connected with these, they can have problems with self-esteem and esthetical appearance (van Berlo et al., 2007). Chronic pain, fatigue and the psychological response to chronic disease like depression and low self-esteem can reduce sexual interest in patients and thereby reduce the frequency as well as the pleasure of intercourse. Several researches have addressed sexual functioning in patients with rheumatic diseases compared to healthy controls. One study investigated the influence of arthritis upon sexual satisfaction and activity by interviewing 169 patients with arthritis and 130 controls. Patients differed from controls in their greater loss of sexual satisfaction over time (Blake, Maisiak, Graciela, Howard, & Brown, 1987).

In previous studies, the prevalence of between 31-76% arthritic patients who experience sexual problems have been reported (Blake et al., 1988; Brown, Dare, Smith, & Meyers; Hill, Herstein, & Walters, 1977; Kraaimaat, Bakker, Janssen, & Bijlsma, 1996). In most studies, subjective interviews or self-constructed/self-reported questionnaires have been used (i.e., Dorner et al., 2018). Furthermore, studies considerably carried out a difference by means of the method preferred, with only a few using healthy controls (Blake et al., 1987; 1988; Curry, Levine, Corty, Jones, & Kurit, 1994).

In another study, half of the patients with rheumatoid arthritis (RA) lost sexual interest during their disease and 60% of them were unsatisfied with their sexual quality of life (Hill, Bird, & Thorpe, 2003).

Sexual dysfunctions are equally experienced by male and female patients. Physical disability, pain, and depression were found related to an impaired sex life in 102 male and 118 female RA patients who were living with a spouse (Kraaimaat et al., 1996).

By contrast, in the younger age group and in patients with inactive or less active disease, sexual activity and frequency of intercourse was not different from healthy, age-matched controls as in a study of 126 women and 35 men with a history of juvenile chronic arthritis (JCA; Østensen, Almberg, & Koksvik, 2000).

Rheumatic diseases can impair also male fertility by direct involvement of the gonads, by disturbances of the hypophyseal gonadal hormonal balance and by autoantibodies to testicular cells. Periods of impotence occur in patients with rheumatic disease. Hypoandrogenicity with low levels of testosterone has been found in men with RA, especially in the presence of high disease activity (Packham & Hall, 2002).

Sexual problems in RA could be attributed to physical and psychological variables. Physical variables include difficulties in performing sexual intercourse (sexual disability), while psychological variables include depression, altered body image, worries about partner interest and diminished sexual drive reflected in both diminished desire and satisfaction (Blake et al., 1987; 1988; Ehrlich, 1983; van Lankveld, Ruiterkamp, Näring, & de Rooij, 2004; Josefsson & Gard, 2010). Difficulty in assuming certain positions when hip or knee movements are limited, dyspareunia due to vaginal dryness in secondary Sjogren's syndrome, and joint pain and fatigue during intercourse are the principal manifestations of sexual disability; the latter is experienced by 50%-61% of RA patients (Blake et al., 1987; Bhadauria et al., 1995; Yoshino & Uchida, 1981).

Bermas, Tucker, Winkelman, and Katz (2000), in a cross-sectional survey of 79 persons with RA and 78 spouses, correlated their marital satisfaction. They found that patients and spouses were generally satisfied with their marriages. Moreover, it was showed that lower marital satisfaction in patients was associated with higher education level, patient's greater use of escape into fantasy, patient's greater use of finding blame, and spouse's higher use of escape into fantasy. Spouses less satisfied with their marriages were more likely to use passive acceptance and less likely to find blame. Female spouses were less likely to be satisfied in their marriages than male spouses. They concluded that certain passive coping styles, more highly educated patients and female spouses are associated with lower marital satisfaction in persons with RA and their spouses. Kraaimaat et al., (1996) studied whether physical disability, pain, depressive mood, and criticism by the spouse are differentially related to intrusiveness of RA on sexuality in male and female patients. They found that physical disability, pain, and, to a lesser extent, depression were found to contribute to intrusiveness of RA on sexuality. However, female patients, compared with male patients, appeared to have lower levels of mobility and self-care. They suggested that differences in sexual motivation between men and women might have been influential in the absence of gender differences in intrusiveness.

One of the most important issues about the treatment of sexual dysfunction associated to RA is the fact that neither the sexual functioning is routinely addressed by physicians or health professionals, nor is it part of frequently used questionnaires to assess physical function or quality of life (Tristano, 2014).

2.2. Systemic Lupus Eryhematosus

Systemic lupus erythematosus (SLE) is a chronic, complicated, autoimmune disease with cumulative involvement of different organs. Due to unknown reasons, SLE is now 10 times more prevalent in developed countries (Moghadam et al., 2019).

Systemic lupus erythematosus affects all organs and has marked physiological, mental, and cognitive impacts on the patients. It results in sexual and physical dysfunction, depression, and decreased self-confidence (Yin et al., 2017). It increases stress and depression by 5–80% in female patients (Kartoz, 2015). A study by Morales et al., (2013) in Spain showed that persistent pain and fatigue related to SLE could hinder physical and emotional aspects of a sexual relationship. The authors found that the rate of avoiding a sexual relationship was higher (50%) and the rates of desire, arousal, lubrication, and orgasm were lower in patients with SLE. Sexual dysfunctions in these patients are associated with physical complaints, obsessive-compulsive symptoms, interpersonal sensitivity, psychoticism, decreased vitality, and impaired social function and mental health (Bachen, Chesney, & Criswell, 2009; Quinzanos et al., 2015).

In a Chinese study, Shen et al., (2015) found that 64% of the SLE patients had impaired sexual function. The authors emphasized that age, marital status, depression, and body image disturbances were the strongest predictors of impaired sexual function in SLE patients.

Moreover, literature (Knight, Vickery, & Fiksand Barg, 2016; McElhone, Abbott, Gray, Williams, & Teh, 2010) reported that fatigue was a global SLE symptom resulting in marital and family problems through causing sexual, physical, mental, and psychological dysfunction. They found that SLE decreased all aspects (physical, sexual, mental, and social) of the quality of life of female patients. Gonadal and sexual dysfunction has been found at an increased rate in men with SLE (Gordon, Beastall, Thomson, & Sturrock, 1988). Decreased libido, erectile dysfunction and failure to ejaculate has been reported in 19-35% of men with SLE (Silva et al., 2009).

2.3. Idiopathic Inflammatory Myopathies

Idiopathic inflammatory myopathies (IIM), such as dermatomyositis (DM), juvenile dermatomyositis (JDM), and polymyositis (PM), are systemic autoimmune disorders characterized by chronic muscular inflammation and progressive muscular weakness.

The annual incidence of IIM ranges from 0.5 to 8.4 cases per one million people, with higher frequency in two age groups (10 to 15 years and 45 to 64 years), affecting more females than males (Feldman, Rider, Reed, & Pachman, 2008; Sallum et al., 2006).

A study (de Souza et al., 2017) demonstrates that the sexual function assessed both by Female Sexual Quotient (FSQ) and Female Sexual Function Index (FSFI) in women with dermatomyositis (DM) and polymyositis (PM) with stable disease was significantly compromised. With respect to FSFI, patients had worse scores in all sub-items (sexual desire, sexual arousal, vaginal lubrication, orgasm, and sexual satisfaction). In addition, patients had significantly more dyspareunia vs. the control group. Sexual dysfunction in patients analyzed in this study was not related to any demographic variable, or to the presence of gynecologic changes.

Reproductive health has not been well studied in male patients with inflammatory myopathies (IIM). In a study, however, testicular morphology and function as well as sexual function in men with IIM are investigated in detail (Silva et al., 2009). Comparing reproductive health of 25 men with IIM to 25 healthy men studied by the same methods showed significantly impaired sexual activity and fertility in patients. Of concern was the significant increase of testicular atrophy in men with IIM and of abnormal semen morphology. Damage to gonadal tissue did impair fertility in these patients. Long disease duration and older age was associated with erectile dysfunction in patients with IIM whereas disease activity and treatment or hypogonadism did not influence it. Again, the latter finding points to psychological problems arising during a chronic disease course over years. The impact of rheumatic disease on sexual functioning is not routinely addressed by physicians or health professionals, nor it is part of frequently used questionnaires to assess physical function or quality of life. The neglect of this important area prevents adequate counselling and intervention. Clarifying the impact of both physical and mental factors on sexuality will help patients to improve quality of life, even when living with a chronic rheumatic disease (Østensen, 2009; 2017).

To conclude, reproductive health and gonadal function are compromised in men with IIM. Patient care should include a discussion on sexuality and contraception, prevention of sexually transmissible diseases, teratogenicity of some drugs used in the treatment, as well as awareness of the risks of the disease and medication represent to fertility (Silva et al., 2009).

Dysfunction and reduction of the sexual activity, such as observed in IIM patients in this study, have been described in male populations with chronic rheumatic diseases, especially rheumatoid arthritis (Helland, Dagfinrud & Kvien, 2008), ankylosing spondylitis (Dincer, Cakar, Kiralp, & Dursun, 2007), and SLE (Stein, Walters, Dillon, & Schulzer, 1986; Folomeev, Alekberova, 1990).

A multidisciplinary approach is essential for patients with idiopathic inflammatory myopathies, in order to provide prevention and care for their sexual life, providing a better quality of life both for these patients and their partners (de Souza et al., 2017).

2.4. Sjögren's Syndrome

Primary Sjögren's syndrome (pSS) is the second most common systemic autoimmune disease, with a female: male ratio of 9:1 (Fox, 2005). pSS is characterized by sicca symptoms of the eyes and mouth and other extra glandular symptoms like arthritis and fatigue. Moreover, women with pSS report often vaginal dryness and dyspareunia (Cirpan et al., 2007; Haga,

Gjesdal, Irgens, & Ostensen, 2005), with negative effects on sexual function, quality of life (Al-Ezzi, Pathak, Tappuni & Khan, 2017) and sexual satisfaction (Isik et al., 2017). Chronic dyspareunia can also be present (Mulherin et al., 1997). Of all sicca symptoms in pSS, vaginal dryness has emerged to have the greatest impact on quality of life (Belenguer et al., 2005). The pathogenesis of vaginal dryness in pSS is not known, but a study has suggesting local inflammation of the vaginal mucosa as a possible explanation (Skopouli, Papanikolaou, Malamou-Mitsi, Papanikolaou, & Moutsopoulos, 1994). Dyspareunia and vaginal dryness can represent an extra barrier to the enjoyment of sexual activity (Tristano, 2009). More recently, Maddali Bongi, Del Rosso, Orlandi, and Matucci-Cerinic (2013) found that more than half of their patients with pSS rated sexual activity as important. However, 68% of the patients reported an interference of pSS symptoms on their sexual life, especially reduced libido, vaginal or vulvar dryness and dyspareunia. Moreover, depression related to sexual dysfunction in these patients (van Nimwegen et al., 2015).

3. Caregiver Burden in Rheumatic Autoimmune Disease

Many factors connected to rheumatic autoimmune diseases, such as chronic inflammatory pattern of pain, long duration of morning stiffness, development of hand deformities or dysfunctions as the disease progresses, nocturnal pain, and difficulty in mobility may cause these patients to become dependent on other people. In fact, patients with a history of onset of more than five years were reported to seriously need help from others, especially in household tasks. The people responsible for the care of patients are called caregivers, who undertake a very critical task for the patient due to the mentioned nature and characteristics of the disease. They also remain under pressure with the sustained course and ongoing requirements of the disease. All these factors challenge caregivers in many aspects such as physical and psychological strain, restriction in social life, and feeling of need for family support, disturbed sleep, financial problems, time constraint, and accompaniment of their own diseases, which collectively create an overloading on caregivers (Sabaz Karakeci, Çetintaş, & Kaya, 2017). Tension, burden, and feeling of loneliness with depressive mood are common features of caregivers, particularly when they are family members of the affected individual. If untreated, these may lead to physical impairment and mental deterioration (Goode, Haley, Roth, & Ford, 1998).

The concept of caregiver burden has been investigated widely, both in general and among caregivers of specific groups of patients (i.e., Eleuteri, Bellanti, & Falaschi, 2016; Simonelli et al., 2008). Studies in this field reveal that caring for an individual with disability is burdensome and stressful, which contributes to lower quality of life, psychiatric morbidity and early mortality of the caregiver (Schulz & Beach, 1999).

Previous studies have investigated variables that could explain or predict the burden as perceived by caregivers. It has been shown that caregiver burden can be explained or predicted by three types of factor: patient characteristics, caregiver characteristics and objective caregiver burden, e.g., the number of care tasks to perform (Vernooij-Dassen, Persoon, & Felling, 1996).

CONCLUSION

Increased knowledge and awareness of rheumatologists, nurses, and care providers about physical, sexual, and psychological aspects of care plays an important role in improved management of these patients.

Most patients with sexual dysfunction rarely talked about sexual complaints with their rheumatologist. Patients with rheumatic diseases' sexual health is often neglected, with both patients and physicians reporting to find it difficult to address sexual complaints, (van Nimwegen et al., 2015).

Sexual health, in fact, is considered an important aspect of physical and mental health and is associated with general well-being and satisfaction with life (Stephenson & Meston, 2015). Sexual function is influenced by physical and psychological consequences of rheumatic diseases, detailed above (Østensen, 2004; 2017).

A survey on current practice and barriers to the management of sexual issues in rheumatology (Helland, Garratt, Kjeken, Kvien & Dagfinrud, 2013) clearly demonstrate that although sexual issues are considered relevant by nearly all health care professionals (HPs), the majority do not ask about or discuss these issues with patients. When sexually related conversations do occur, the patient is the primary initiator, with HPs failing to take the responsibility to raise the topic of sexuality. The perceived embarrassment of the patient was reported as the most important barrier to raising disease-related sexual issues (83%), followed by lack of time (72%), patient's ethnicity (59%), own knowledge (56%), own embarrassment (52%), patient's age (51%), and lack of privacy (47%). The two factors perceived to be least restrictive for sexually related conversations were patient's marital status (12%) and same gender as patient (5%). Two-thirds (67%) of all respondents reported that they had no education in sexuality, and the majority (71%) stated that specific training was needed. Age, further education in sexual issues, and being comfortable with addressing sexual issues significantly increased the chance of initiating sexual topics in patient consultations, whereas being a physiotherapist (compared to being a nurse) significantly reduced the same chance. The common problem is communication, so an open conversation including inquiry about sexuality in routine care is the first step to improve the situation. To allow the patients to present problems and concerns without embarrassment is also important. After an open discussion is achieved, the treatment will depend on the specific patient's symptoms. Knowledge and openness concerning sexual issues need to be emphasized as part of the competence of health professionals (Helland, Kjeken, Steen, Kvien, Hauge, & Dagfinrud, 2011).

There are some general recommendations including: discussion of the problems with the partner, principally about the partner's fear in causing pain or distress during sexual intercourse; exploring different positions; using analgesic drugs, heat, and muscle relaxants before sexual activity in order to decrease pain; exploring alternative methods of sexual expression; and physiotherapy (Panush et al., 2000; Tristano, 2009).

The literature focused on the sexual problems in these patients stress that sexual problems could have an impact on relational aspects in patients with a partner. We therefore, suggest, in single patients, to assess sexual life and to explain repercussion of these disease on sexual life, suggesting practical solutions that could solve or decrease the problem. In patients with a partner, assess if there is a sexual problem, and, if there is, try to understand if there are relational problems to investigate and to solve.

A multidisciplinary approach is therefore essential, in order to provide prevention and care for their sexual life, providing a better quality of life both for these patients and their partners (de Souza et al., 2017).

A recent study (Helland, Dagfinrud, Haugen, Kjeken, & Zangi, 2017) underlined the need for including sexual issues in the care and rehabilitation of patients with rheumatic diseases. Patients want HPs to know about the possible challenges posed by these diseases in terms of patients' sex lives and intimate relationships, and to facilitate communication about these aspects. Therefore, there is a need for developing practice guidelines to integrate sexuality as an aspect of healthcare delivery in a patient-friendly manner. The findings indicate the various potential benefits of HPs' inclusion of sexual issues in their dialogue with patients, and the need of incorporating these topics in HPs' training (Helland et al., 2013).

References

Abdel-Nasser, A. M., & Ali, E. I. (2006). Determinants of sexual disability and dissatisfaction in female patients with rheumatoid arthritis. *Clinical Rheumatology*, 25, 822-830. doi: 10.1007/s10067-005-0175-0.

Al-Ezzi, M. Y., Pathak, N., Tappuni, A. R. & Khan, K. S. (2017). Primary Sjögren's syndrome impact on smell, taste, sexuality and quality of life in female patients: A systematic review and meta-analysis. *Modern Rheumatology*, 27, 623-629. doi: 10.1080/14397595.2016.1249538.

Aras, H., Aras, B., Icagasioglu, A., Yumusakhuylu, Y., Kemahli, E., Haliloglu, S., & Oguz, F. M. (2013). Sexual dysfunction in women with rheumatoid arthritis. *Medicinski Glasnik,* 10(2), 327-331.

Bachen, E. A., Chesney, M. A., & Criswell, L. A. (2009). Prevalence of mood and anxiety disorders in women with systemic lupus erythematosus. *Arthritis Care & Research*, 61, 822-829. doi: 10.1002/art.24519.

Belenguer, R., Ramos-Casals, M., Brito-Zerón, P., del Pino, J., Sentís, J., Aguiló, S., & Font J. (2005). Influence of clinical and immunological parameters on the health-related quality of life of patients with primary Sjögren's syndrome. *Clinical & Experimental Rheumatology*, 23(3):351-6.

Bermas, B. L., Tucker, J. S., Winkelman, D. K., & Katz, J. N. (2000). Marital satisfaction in couples with rheumatoid arthritis. *Arthritis Care & Research*, 13, 149-155.

Bhadauria, S., Moser, D. K., Clements, P. J., Singh, R. R., Lachenbruch, P. A., Pitkin, R. M., & Weiner, S. R. (1995). Genital tract abnormalities and female sexual function impairment in systemic sclerosis. *American Journal of Obstetrics and Gynecology*, 172, 580-587. doi: 10.1016/0002-9378(95)90576-6.

Blake, D. J., Maisiak, R., Graciela, S., Howard, L.H., & Brown, S. (1987). Sexual quality of life of patients with arthritis compared to arthritis free controls. *Journal of Rheumatology*, 14, 570–576.

Blake, D. J., Maisiak, R., Koplan, A., Alarcón, G. S., & Brown, S. (1988). Sexual dysfunction among patients with arthritis. *Clinical Rheumatology,* 7, 50-60. doi: 10.1007/BF02284057.

Brown, G. M. M., Dare, C. M., Smith, P. R., & Meyers, O. L. (1987). Important problems identified by patients with chronic arthritis. *South African Medical Journal*, 72, 126–128.

Carmona, L., Cross, M., Williams, B., Lassere, M., & March, L. (2010). Rheumatoid arthritis. *Best Practice & Research: Clinical Rheumatology*, 24, 733-745. doi: 10.1016/j.berh.2010.10.001.

Cirpan, T., Guliyeva, A., Onder, G., Terek, M. C., Ozsaran, A., Kabasakal, Y., Yucebilgin, S. (2007). Comparison of human papillomavirus testing and cervical cytology with colposcopic examination and biopsy in cervical cancer screening in a cohort of patients with Sjogren's syndrome. *European Journal of Gynaecological Oncology*, 28, 302-306.

Coskun, B., Coskun, B. N., Atis, G., Ergenekon, E., Dilek, K. (2013). Evaluation of Sexual Function in Women with Rheumatoid Arthritis. *Urology Journal,* 10, 1081-1087.

Curry, S. L., Levine, S. B., Corty, E., Jones, P. K., Kurit, D. M. (1994). The impact of systemic lupus erythematosuson women's sexual functioning. *Journal of Rheumatology*, 21, 2254–2260.

de Souza, F. H. C, Brito de Araújo, D., Silvad, C. A., Miossi, R., Najjar Abdoe, C. H., Bonfáf, E., & Katsuyuki Shinjo, S. (2017). Analysis of sexual function of patients with dermatomyositis and polymyositis through self-administered questionnaires: a cross-sectional study. *Revista Brasileira de Rheumatologia,* 57, 134-140. doi: 10.1016/j.rbre. 2016.11.002.

Dincer, U., Cakar, E., Kiralp, M. Z., & Dursun, H. (2007). Assessment of sexual dysfunction in male patients with Ankylosing Spondylitis. *Rheumatology International*, 27, 561-566. doi: 10.1007%2Fs00296-006-0248-7.

Dorner, T. E., Berner, C., Haider, S., Grabovac, I., Lamprecht, T., Fenzl, K. H., Erlacher, L. (2018). Sexual health in patients with rheumatoid arthritis and the association between physical fitness and sexual function: a cross-sectional study. *Rheumatology International*, 38, 1103–1114. doi: 10.1007/s00296-018-4023-3.

Ehrlich, G. E. (1983). Social, economic, psychologic and sexual outcomes in rheumatoid arthritis. *American Journal of Medicine*, 75, 27–34. doi: 10.1016/0002-9343(83)90472-2.

Eleuteri, S., Bellanti, G., & Falaschi, P. (2016). Hip fracture: preliminary results supporting significative correlations between the psychological wellbeing of patients and their relative caregivers. *Journal of Gerontology and Geriatrics*, 64, 104-111.

Eleuteri, S., Rossi, R., & Simonelli, C. (2019). How to address clinical work with older bisexual clients and their partners? *Sexologies*, 28, e36-e43. doi: 10.1016/j.sexol.2019.05.0109.

Feldman, B. M., Rider, L. G., Reed, A. M., & Pachman, L. M. (2008). Juvenile dermatomyositis and other idiopathic inflammatory myopathies of childhood. *Lancet*, 371, 2201-2012.

Folomeev, M., & Alekberova, Z. (1990). Impotence in systemic lupus erythematosus. *Journal of Rheumatology*, 17, 117-119.

Fox, R. I. (2005). Sjogren's syndrome. *Lancet*, 366, 321-331. doi: 10.1016/S0140-6736(05)66990-5.

Frikha, F., Maazoun, F., Salah, R. B., Snoussi, M., Masmoudi, J., Nabil Mhiri, M., & Bahloul, Z. (2011). Sexual Function in Married Women with Rheumatoid Arthritis. *Presse Medicale*, 40 (12 Pt 1), e521-e527.

Goldblatt, F., & O'Neill, S. G. (2013). Clinical aspects of autoimmune rheumatic diseases. *Lancet,* 382, 797-808. doi: 10.1016/S0140-6736 (13)61499-3.

Goode, K. T., Haley, W. E., Roth, D. L., & Ford, G. R. (1998). Predictinglongitudinal changes in caregiver physical and mentalhealth: a stress process model. *Health Psychology*, 17, 190-8. doi:10.1037/ 0278-6133.17.2.190.

Gordon, D., Beastall, G. H., Thomson, J. A., & Sturrock, R. D. (1988). Prolongedhypogonadism in male patients with rheumatoid arthritis duringflares in disease activity. *Revista Brasileira de Rheumatologia*, 27, 440-444.doi: 10.1093/rheumatology/27.6.440.

Haga, H. J., Gjesdal, C. G., Irgens, L. M., & Ostensen, M. (2005). Reproduction and gynaecological manifestations inwomen with primary Sjogren's syndrome: a case-controlstudy. *Scandinavian Journal of Rheumatology*, 34, 45-48.doi: 10.1080/03009740510017959.

Helland, Y., Dagfinrud, H., Haugen, M., Kjeken, I., & Zangi, H. (2017). Patients' Perspectives on Information and Communication About Sexual and Relational Issues in Rheumatology Health Care. *Musculoskeletal Care* 15, 131–139.

Helland, Y., Dagfinrud, H., & Kvien, T. K. (2008). Perceived influence of health status on sexual activity in RA patients: associations with demographic and disease-related variables. *Scandinavian Journal of Rheumatology*, 37, 194-199. doi: 10.1080/03009740701867349.

Helland, Y., Garratt, A., Kjeken, I., Kvien, T. K., & Dagfinrud, H. (2013) Current practice and barriers to the management of sexual issues in rheumatology: results of a survey of health professionals, *Scandinavian Journal of Rheumatology*, 42 (1), 20-26.doi: 10.3109/03009742.2012.709274.

Helland, Y., Kjeken, I, Steen, E., Kvien, T. K., Hauge, M., & Dagfinrud, H. (2011). Rheumatic Diseases and Sexuality: Disease Impact and Self-Management Strategies. *Arthritis Care & Research*, 63 (5), 743-50. doi: 10.1002/acr.20424.

Hill, J., Bird, H., & Thorpe, R. (2003). Effects of rheumatoid arthritis on sexual activity and relationships. *Rheumatology*, 42, 280-286. doi: 10.1093/rheumatology/keg079.

Hill, R. H., Herstein, A., & Walters, K. (1977). Juvenile rheumatoid arthritis: follow-up into adulthood-medical, sexual and social status. *Canadian Medical Association Journal*, 114, 790–794.

Isik H., Isik, M., Aynioglua, O., Karcaaltincabad, N., Sahbaza, A., Beyazciceke, T., & Demircane, N. (2017). Are the women with Sjögren's Syndrome satisfied with their sexual activity? *Revista Brasileira de Rheumatologia*, 57(3), 210–216.

Jacobi, C. E., Triemstra, M., Rupp, I., Dinant, H. J., & Van Den Bos, G. A. (2001). Health care utilization among rheumatoid arthritispatients referred to a rheumatology center: unequal needs, unequal care? *Arthritis & Rheumatology*, 45, 324–30. doi: 10.1002/1529-0131(200108)45:4<324::AID-ART344>3.0.CO;2-1.

Jacobi, C. E., van den Berg, B., Boshuizen, H. C., Rupp, I., Dinant, H. J., & van den Bos, G. A. (2003). Dimension-specific burden of caregiving amongpartners of rheumatoid arthritis patients. *Rheumatology*, 42, 1226–1233. doi:10.1093/rheumatology/keg366.

Josefsson, K. A., & Gard, G. (2010). Women's Experiences of Sexual Health When Living With Rheumatoid Arthritis--An Explorative Qualitative Study. *BMC Musculoskeletal Disorders*.11, 240. doi: 10.1186/1471-2474-11-240.

Josefsson, K. A., & Gard, G. (2012). Sexual Health in Patients with Rheumatoid Arthritis: Experiences, Needs and Communication with Health Care Professionals. *Musculoskeletal Care*, 10 (2), 76-89.

Kartoz, C. R. (2015). Reproductive Health Concerns in Women with Systemic Lupus Erythematosus. *MCN: The American Journal of Maternal/Child Nursing*, 40, 220-226.doi: 10.1097/NMC.000000 0000000145.

Klippel, J. H., & Dieppe, P. A. (1998). *Rheumatology*. 2nd edn. London: Mosby International, 1998.

Knight, A., Vickery, M., Fiks, A., & Barg, F. K. (2016). The illness experience of youth with lupus/mixed connective tissue disease: a mixed methods analysis of patient and parent perspectives. *Lupus*, 25, 1028-1039. doi: 10.1177/0961203316646460.

Kraaimaat, F. W., Bakker, A. H., Janssen, E., & Bijlsma, J. W. (1996). Intrusiveness of rheumatoid arthritis on sexuality in male and female patients living with a spouse. *Arthritis Care & Research*, 9, 120–125. doi: 10.1002/1529-0131(199604)9:2<120::AID-ANR1790090208>3.0. CO;2-T.

Lindqvist, E., Saxne, T., Geborek, P., & Eberhardt, K. (2002). Ten yearoutcome in a cohort of patients with early rheumatoidarthritis: health status, disease process, and damage. *Annals of the Rheumatic Diseases*, 61, 1055–9.

Lipsky, P. E. (2005). Rheumatoid Arthritis. In D. L. Kasper, E. Braunwald, A. S. Fauci, S. L. Hauser, D. L. Longo, & J. L. Jameson (Eds.), *Harrison's Principles of Internal Medicine* (pp. 1968-1977). New York: McGraw-Hill.

Maddali Bongi, S, Del Rosso, A, Orlandi, M, & Matucci-Cerinic, M. (2013). Gynaecological symptoms and sexual disabilityin women with primary Sjögren's syndrome and siccasyndrome. *Clinical and Experimental Rheumatology*, 31, 683-690.

McElhone, K., Abbott, J., Gray, J., Williams, A., & Teh, L. S. (2010). Patient perspective ofsystemic lupus erythematosus in relation to health-related quality of life concepts: a qualitative study. *Lupus*, 19, 1640-1647.doi: 10.1177/0961203310378668.

Moghadam, Z. B., Rezaei, E., Faezi, S. T., Zareian, A., Ibrahim, F. M., & Ibrahim, M. M. (2019). Prevalence of sexual dysfunction in women with systemic lupus erythematosus and its related factors. *Reumatologia*, 57, 19-26. doi: 10.5114/reum.2019.83235.

Morales, M. G., Rubio, J. C., Peralta-Ramírez, M., Romero, L. J., Fernández, R. R., Camps García, M. T., Centeno, N. O. (2013). Impaired sexual function in women with systemic lupus erythematosus: a cross-sectional study. *Lupus*, 22, 987-995.doi: 10.1177/0961203313500370.

Mulherin, D. M., Sheeran, T. P., Kumararatne, D. S., Speculand, B., Luesley, D., & Situnayake, R. D. (1997). Sjögren's syndrome in women presenting with chronicdyspareunia. *British Journal of Obstetrics and Gynaecology,* 104, 1019-23.doi: 10.1111/j.1471-0528.1997.tb12060.x.

Østensen, M. (2004). New insights into sexual functioning andfertility in rheumatic diseases. *Best Practice & Research: Clinical Rheumatology,* 18, 21-32.doi:10.1016/j.berh.2004.01.002.

Østensen, M. (2009). Sexual functioning is impaired in patients with rheumatic disease independent of disease activity, therapy or gonadal function. *Revista Brasileira de Rheumatologia,* 49(6), 639-642. doi: 10.1590/S0482-50042009000600001.

Østensen, M. (2017). Sexual and reproductivehealth in rheumaticdisease. *Nature Reviews Rheumatology*, 13, 485–493. doi: 10.1038/nrrheum. 2017.102.

Østensen, M., Almberg, K., & Koksvik, H.S. (2000). Sex, reproduction, andgynecological disease in young adults with a history of juvenilechronic arthritis. *Journal of Rheumatology*, 27, 1783-1787.

Packham, J. C., & Hall, M. A. (2002). Longterm follow-up of 246 adults withjuvenile idiopathic arthritis: social function, relationships and sexualactivity. *Rheumatology*, 41, 440-443.doi: 10.1093/rheumatology/ 41.12.1440.

Panush, R. S., Mihailescu, G. D., Gornisiewicz, M. T., & Sutaria, S. H. (2000). Sex andarthritis. *Bulletin on the Rheumatic Diseases*, 49, 1-4.

Pirildar, T., Müezzinoğlu, T., & Pirildar, S. (2004). Sexual function in ankylosing spondylitis: a study of 65 men. *Journal of Urology*, 171, 1598-1600doi: 10.1097/01.ju.0000117867.44858.ba.

Quinzanos, I., Davis, L., Keniston, A., Nash, A., Yazdany, J., Fransen, R., and Zell, J. (2015). Application and feasibility of systemic lupus erythematosus reproductive health care quality indicators at a public urban rheumatology clinic. *Lupus*, 24,203-209. doi: 10.1177/096120 3314552832.

Revenson, T. A., & Majerovitz, S. D. (1991). The effects of chronic illness on the spouse. Social resources as stress buffers. *Arthritis Care & Research*, 4, 63–72.

SabazKarakeci, E., Çetintaş, D., & Kaya, A. (2017). Association of the Commitments and Responsibilities of the Caregiver within the Family to the Disease Activity in Patients with Rheumatoid Arthritis: A Report from Turkey. *Archives of rheumatology*, *33*(2), 213–220. doi:10.5606/ ArchRheumatol.2018.6427.

Sallum, A. M., Kiss, M. H. B., Silva, C. A., Wakamatsu, A. M. A. A. G., Vianna, M. A. A. G., Sachetti, S., & Marie, S. K. N. (2006). Difference in adhesion molecule expression (ICAM-1 and VCAM-1) in juvenile and adult dermatomyositis, polymyositis and inclusion body myositis. *Autoimmunity Reviews*, 5, 93-100. doi: 10.1016/j.autrev.2005.05.008.

Schulz, R., & Beach, S. R. (1999). Caregiving as a risk factor formortality: the Caregiver Health Effects Study. *Journal of the American Medical Association*, 282, 2215–2219.doi: 10.1001/jama.282.23.2215.

Shen, B., He, Y., Chen, H., Zhao, C., Zhu, L., Gao, Y., and Liu, J. (2015). Body Image Disturbances Have Impact on the Sexual Problems in Chinese Systemic Lupus Erythematosus Patients. *Journal of Immunology Research*, 2015, 204513. doi: 10.1155/2015/204513.

Silva, C. A., Febrônio, M. V., Bonfá, E., Rodrigues Pereira, R. M., de Pereira, E. A. G., & Duarte Takiuiti, A. (2009). Sexual function and reproductive health in adolescent females with systemic lupus erythematosus. *Revista Brasileira de Rheumatologia*, 49, 690-702. doi: 10.1590/S0482-50042009000600006.

Silva, C. A., de Moraes, A. J. P., Leal, M. M. M., Sallum, A. M. E., Bonfá, E., Borges, C. T. L, Hallak, J. (2009). Reproductive health aspects in men with idiopathic inflammatory myopathy. A multicenter study.

Revista Brasileira de Rheumatologia, 49, 677-689. doi: 10.1590/ S0482-50042009000600005.

Simonelli, C., Tripodi, F., Rossi, R., Fabrizi, A., Lembo, D., Cosmi, V., & Pierleoni, L The influence of caregiver burden on sexual intimacy andmarital satisfaction in couples with an Alzheimer spouse. *International Journal of Clinical Practice*, 62 (1), 47–52. doi: 10.1111/j.1742-1241.2007.01506.x.

Skopouli, F. N., Papanikolaou, S., Malamou-Mitsi, V., Papanikolaou, N., & Moutsopoulos, H. M. (1994). Obstetric and gynaecological profile in patients with primary Sjögren'ssyndrome. *Annals of the Rheumatic Disease*, 53:569-573.doi: 10.1136/ard.53.9.569.

Stein, H., Walters, K., Dillon, A., & Schulzer, M. (1986). Systemic lupus erythematosus – a medical and social profile. *Journal of Rheumatology*, 13, 570-575.

Stephenson, K. R., & Meston, C. M. (2015). The conditional importance of sex: exploring the association between sexual wellbeing and life satisfaction. *Journal of Sex and Marital Therapy*, 41, 25-38. doi: 10.1080/0092623X.2013.811450.

Tavares Queiroz de Almeidaa, P. H., de Castro Ferreirac, C., Shu Kurizkyb, P., FeitosaMunizd, L., & da Motab, L. M. H. (2015). How the rheumatologist can guide the patient with rheumatoid arthritis on sexual function. *Revista Brasileira de Rheumatologia*, 55, 458-463. doi: 10.1016/j.rbre.2016.11.002.

Træen, B., Štulhofer A., Janssen, E., Carvalheira, A. A., Hald, G. M., Lange, T., & Graham, C., (2019). Sexual Activity and Sexual Satisfaction among Older Adults in Four European Countries. *Archives of Sexual Behavior, 48* (3), 815-829. doi: 10.1007/s10508-018-1256-x.

Tristano, A. G. (2009). The impact of rheumatic diseases on sexual function. *Rheumatology International*, 29, 853-860. doi: 10.1007/s00296-009-0850-6.

Tristano, A. G. (2014). Impact of rheumatoid arthritis on sexual function. *World Journal of Orthopedics*, 18, 5, 107-111. doi: 10.5312/wjo.v5. i2.107.

van Berlo, W. T., van de Wiel, H. B., Taal, E., Rasker, J. J.,Weijmar Schultz, W. C., & van Rijswijk, M. H. (2007). Sexual functioning of people with rheumatoid arthritis: a multicenter study. *Clinical Rheumatology*, 26, 30-38.doi:10.1007/s10067-006-0216-3.

van Lankveld, W., Ruiterkamp, G., Näring, G., & de Rooij, DJ. (2004). Marital and sexual satisfaction in patients with RA and their spouses. *Scandinavian Journal of Rheumatology*, 33, 405-408.doi: 10.1080/03009740410010317.

van Nimwegen, J. F., Arends, S., van Zuiden, G. S., Vissink, A., Kroese, F. G. M., & Bootsma, H. (2015). The impact of primary Sjögren's syndrome on female sexual function. *Rheumatology*, 54, 1286-1293. doi:10.1093/rheumatology/keu522.

Vernooij-Dassen, M. J. F. J., Persoon, J. M. G., & Felling, A. J. A. (1996). Predictors of sense of competence in caregivers of demented persons. *Social Science & Medicine*, 43, 41–49.doi: 10.1016/0277-9536(95)00332-0.

Yildiz, C., Karakus, S., BozokluAkkar, O., Sahin, A., Bozkurt, B., & Yanik, A. (2017). Primary Sjögren's Syndrome Adversely Affects the Female Sexual Function Assessed by the Female Sexual Function Index: A Case-Control Study. *Archives of rheumatology*, 32(2), 123-128. doi: 10.5606/ArchRheumatol.2017.6066.

Yin, R., Xu, B., Li, L., Fu, T., Zhang, L., Zhang, Q., Shen, B. (2017). The impact of systemic lupus erythematosus on women's sexual functioning. A systematic review and meta-analysis. *Medicine* 96 (27), e7162. doi: 10.1097/MD.0000000000007162.

Yoshino, S., & Uchida, S. (1981). Sexual problems of women with rheumatoid arthritis. *Archives of Physical Medicine and Rehabilitation*, 62, 122–123.

Zhang, Q., Zhou, C., Chen, H., Zhao, Q., Li, L., Cui, Y., & Shen, B. (2018). Rheumatoid arthritis is associated with negatively variable impacts on domainsof female sexual function: Evidence from a systematic review and meta-analysis. *Psychology, Health & Medicine*, 23(1), 114-125. doi: 10.1080/13548506.2017.1338738.

About the Editor

Stefano Eleuteri, PhD
Research Fellow
Department of Psychology
Sapienza University of Rome, Rome, Italy

Psychologist, Psychotherapist, PhD in Social, Developmental Psychology and Educational Research. He is the Deputy Chair of the Education Committee of the Fragility Fracture Network. Since 2010, he works as a psychologist and psychotherapist as a private consultant, also organizing events about psychogeriatrics. Research Fellow at Sapienza University of Rome. Since 2012 he teaches different aspects of psychogeriatrics (Caregiving, Sex & Aging, Psychology of the Elderly) in different higher education courses for nurses and medical doctors at Sapienza University of Rome.

He has been a speaker in the most important local and international congresses in the psychogeriatrics field. He is author of scientific and educational contributions in the psychogeriatrics area, also in indexed journals.

INDEX

A

B

C

D

E

F

G

H

I

J

K

L

M

W